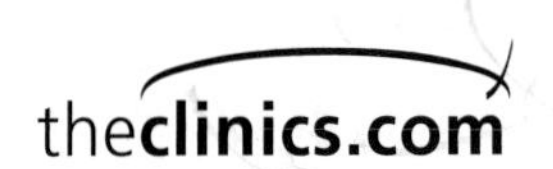

THORACIC SURGERY CLINICS

Ethical Issues in Thoracic Surgery

GUEST EDITOR
Robert M. Sade, MD

CONSULTING EDITOR
Mark K. Ferguson, MD

November 2005 • Volume 15 • Number 4

SAUNDERS

An Imprint of Elsevier, Inc.
PHILADELPHIA LONDON TORONTO MONTREAL SYDNEY TOKYO

W.B. SAUNDERS COMPANY
A Division of Elsevier Inc.

1600 John F. Kennedy Boulevard, Suite 1800 • Philadelphia, Pennsylvania 19103-2899

http://www.theclinics.com

THORACIC SURGERY CLINICS
November 2005
Editor: Catherine Bewick

Volume 15, Number 4
ISSN 1547-4127
ISBN 1-4160-2799-8

Thoracic Surgery Clinics (ISSN 1547-4127) is published quarterly by the W.B. Saunders Company. Corporate and editorial offices: 1600 John F. Kennedy Boulevard, Suite 1800, Philadelphia, PA 19103-2899. Accounting and Circulation Offices: 6277 Sea Harbor Drive, Orlando, FL 32887-4800. Periodicals postage paid at Orlando, FL 32862, and additional mailing offices. Subscription prices are $180.00 per year (US individuals), $270.00 per year (US institutions), $90 per year (US students/individuals), $230.00 per year (Canadian individuals), $335.00 per year (Canadian institutions), $115 per year (Canadian and foreign students/individuals), $230.00 per year (foreign individuals), and $335.00 per year (foreign institutions). Foreign air speed delivery is included in all *Clinics'* subscription prices. All prices are subject to change without notice. POSTMASTER: Send address changes to *Thoracic Surgery Clinics*, W.B. Saunders Company, Periodicals Fulfillment, Orlando, FL 32887-4800. **Customer Service: 1-800-654-2452 (US). From outside of the US, call 1-407-345-4000.** E mail: hhspcs@wbsaunders.com.

Reprints. For copies of 100 or more, of articles in this publication, please contact Commercial Rights Department, Elsevier Inc., 360 Park Avenue South, New York, NY 10010-1710. Tel: (212) 633-3813, Fax: (212) 462-1935, e-mail: reprints@elsevier.com

Thoracic Surgery Clinics is covered in *Index Medicus* and *EMBASE/Excerpta Medica.*

Printed in the United States of America.

CONSULTING EDITOR

MARK K. FERGUSON, MD, Professor of Surgery, Section of Cardiac and Thoracic Surgery, The University of Chicago, Chicago, Illinois

GUEST EDITOR

ROBERT M. SADE, MD, Professor, Department of Surgery, and Director, Institute of Human Values in Health Care, Medical University of South Carolina, Charlestown, South Carolina

CONTRIBUTORS

PETER ANGELOS, MD, PhD, Associate Professor of Surgery, Associate Professor of Medical Humanities and Bioethics, Department of Surgery, Northwestern University, Feinberg School of Medicine, Chicago, Illinois

MARK L. BARR, MD, Associate Professor of Surgery, Department of Cardiothoracic Surgery, University of Southern California; and Childrens Hospital Los Angeles, Los Angeles, California

ANDREW B. COOPER, MD, MHSc, Clinical Assistant Professor, The Interdisciplinary Division of Critical Care Medicine, University of Toronto; and Staff, Sunnybrook and Women's College Health Sciences Centre, Toronto, Ontario, Canada

NEIL J. FARBER, MD, FACP, Chief, General Internal Medicine Faculty, Christiana Care Health System, Wilmington, Delaware; Clinical Professor of Medicine, Thomas Jefferson University, Philadelphia, Pennsylvania

JOHN C. GOODMAN, PhD, National Center for Policy Analysis, Dallas, Texas

DAVID C. GRANT, MD, ARDMS, Department of Emergency Medicine, University of Arizona College of Medicine, Tucson, Arizona

KENNETH V. ISERSON, MD, MBA, FACEP, Department of Emergency Medicine, University of Arizona College of Medicine, Tucson, Arizona

JAY A. JACOBSON, MD, FACP, Professor of Internal Medicine and Chief, Division of Medical Ethics, Department of Internal Medicine, LDS Hospital and University of Utah School of Medicine, Salt Lake City, Utah

JAMES W. JONES, MD, PhD, Montgomery, Texas

LUCIAN L. LEAPE, MD, Adjunct Professor of Health Policy, Harvard School of Public Health, Department of Health Policy and Management, Boston, Massachusetts

K. FRANCIS LEE, MD, MPH, FACS, Department of Surgery, Baystate Medical Center, Tufts University School of Medicine, Springfield, Massachusetts

MARTIN McKNEALLY, MD, PhD, Professor Emeritus, Department of Surgery and Joint Centre for Bioethics, University of Toronto, Toronto, Canada

LAWRENCE B. McCULLOUGH, PhD, Center for Medical Ethics and Health Policy, Baylor College of Medicine, Houston, Texas

FRANKLIN G. MILLER, PhD, Department of Clinical Bioethics, Clinical Center, National Institutes of Health, Bethesda, Maryland

E. HAAVI MORREIM, PhD, Professor, College of Medicine, University of Tennessee Health Science Center, Memphis, Tennessee

SHARON REYNOLDS, RN, BA, BScN, MHSc, Clinical Ethics Fellow, Joint Centre for Bioethics, University of Toronto; Medical-Surgical Intensive Care Unit, Toronto General Hospital, Toronto, Canada

BRUCE W. RICHMAN, MA, Columbia, Missouri

WINFIELD J. WELLS, MD, Associate Professor of Surgery, Department of Cardiothoracic Surgery, University of Southern California; and Childrens Hospital Los Angeles, Los Angeles, California

CONTENTS

Informed consent plays a major role in forming a therapeutic alliance with the patient. The informed consent process has evolved from simple consent, in which the surgeon needed only to obtain the patient's permission for a procedure, into informed consent, in which the surgeon provides the patient with information about clinically salient features of a procedure, the patient understands this information adequately, and the patient voluntarily authorizes the surgeon to perform the procedure. Special circumstances of informed consent include conflicting professional opinions, consent with multiple physicians, patients who are undecided or refuse surgery, patients with diminished decision-making capacity, surrogate decision making, pediatric assent, and consent for the involvement of trainees.

Effective physicians recognize that most patients have difficulty following instructions for a variety of reasons. That difficulty is best understood as nonadherence rather than noncompliance. The surgeon's role is to make the patient's choice informed, to be aware of the risk factors for nonadherence, and not to make adherence any more difficult than it has to be. The patient's role is to make choices between value-laden alternatives. Society's role is to distribute scarce medical resources equitably to patients who can and want to adhere to the necessary regimen to benefit from them.

Withdrawing life-supporting technology from patients who are irremediably ill is morally troubling for caregivers, patients, and families. Interventions that enable clinicians to delay death create situations in which the dignity and comfort of dying patients may be sacrificed to spare professionals and families from their elemental fear of death. Understanding

FORTHCOMING ISSUES

February 2006

Pulmonary Metastases
Robert J. Downey, MD, *Guest Editor*

May 2006

Complications of Esophageal Surgery
Cameron D. Wright, MD, *Guest Editor*

August 2006

Complications of Lung Surgery
Todd L. Demmy, MD, *Guest Editor*

RECENT ISSUES

August 2005

Advances in the Management of Gastroesophageal Reflux Disease
Claude Deschamps, MD, FRCSC, FACS, *Guest Editor*

May 2005

Preoperative Preparation of Patients for Thoracic Surgery
Richard I. Whyte, MD, *Guest Editor*

February 2005

Advances in Anesthesia and Pain Management
Jerome M. Klafta, MD, *Guest Editor*

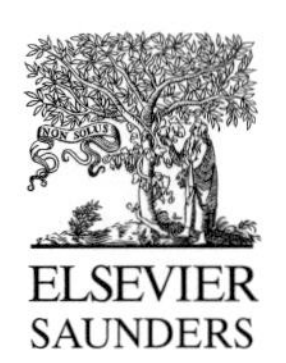

Thorac Surg Clin 15 (2005) xi – xiii

THORACIC
SURGERY
CLINICS

Preface

Ethical Issues in Thoracic Surgery

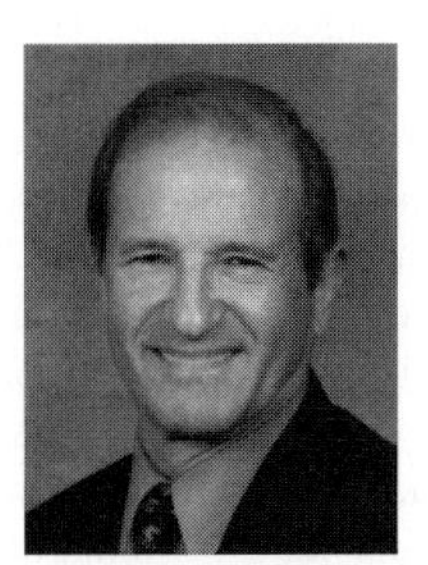

Robert M. Sade, MD
Guest Editor

The Latin expression *primum non nocere* ("above all, do no harm)" is perhaps the most misattributed, misunderstood, and misused expression in medical ethics. It is usually attributed to Hippocrates, yet it appears nowhere in Hippocratic writings. The closest ancient statement is probably "To help, or at least, to do no harm," which appears in the Hippocratic corpus, in Epidemics, Book I, Section XI. The specific phrase *primum non nocere* is, in fact, not of ancient origin at all, but has been attributed to the seventeenth-century physician Thomas Sydenham [1]. The phrase was first used by a surgeon, L.A. Stimson, MD, in the late nineteenth century, and was in common usage by the turn of the century [2].

A more substantial problem with the Latin phrase, however, is that it advocates the impossible. Virtually every medical encounter, diagnostic procedure, or treatment is harmful to a greater or lesser degree. The expression is particularly inappropriate in the context of surgery, because surgical interventions nearly always begin with traumatic injury to the patient in the form of an incision through skin or mucous membrane. A more appropriate aphorism for both surgery and medicine would be: "Above all, do more good than harm." An expression of this kind might be considered by some surgeons to lie at the heart of surgical ethics, but I believe it to be a corollary to the foundation of all medical ethics, as stated in the American Medical Association Code of Medical Ethics: "A physician shall, while caring for a patient, regard responsibility to the patient as paramount" [3].

A recent study compared the surgical with the medical literature, looking at the subject matter of the papers published in 12 surgical and 15 medical journals. The authors found, among many thousands of articles, that substantive discussion of an ethical issue could be identified in 2.7% of articles found in medical journal articles and in only 0.6% of those found in surgical journals; that is, ethical matters were discussed more than four times as often in the medical literature as in the surgical literature [4]. Why do surgeons consider ethical issues less frequently than other physicians in their publications and, presumably in their professional meetings? One well-known surgical educator put it this way: "The difference between surgeons and internists is that surgeons *practice* ethics, while internists mainly *talk* about it" [5].

Regardless of its origins, the gap may be narrowing, at least in cardiothoracic surgery. In recent years, there has been increasing interest in discussing ethical issues in both the CT literature and at CT meetings. Some of this has been due to the efforts of the Ethics Forum, which was established in 1999 for the purpose of encouraging education in ethical issues for cardiothoracic surgery. It comprises members of The Society of Thoracic Surgeons Standards and Ethics Committee and members of The American Associa-

1547-4127/05/$ – see front matter
doi:10.1016/j.thorsurg.2005.07.001

tion for Thoracic Surgery Ethics Committee. From 2000 to 2005, members of the Ethics Forum published 113 articles on ethical topics in the surgery literature, many of which are touched upon in this issue of the *Thoracic Surgery Clinics*.

The issue is divided into three sections: Clinical Ethics and the Surgeon at the Bedside; Bioethics in Health Care Policy; and Biomedical Research Ethics. The section on Clinical Ethics and The Surgeon at the Bedside begins with Jones, McCullough, and Richman discussing consent ("Informed Consent: It's Not Just Signing a Form"). They review the fundamentals of informed consent, how the requirements for consent are best met, and the process of consent under special circumstances, such as compromised or limited capacity to make decisions, dealing with conflicting professional opinions, surrogate decision making, and the flip side of informed consent for surgery: informed refusal.

Jay Jacobson ("The Effect of Patients' Noncompliance on Surgeons' Obligations") explores the circumstances under which surgeons have specific obligations to care for noncompliant patients, as well as suggesting ways to identify such patients and to work with them effectively to make the relationship less onerous.

Reynolds, Cooper, and McNeally ("Withdrawing Life Sustaining Treatment: Ethical Considerations") describe the difficult and morally troublesome aspects of withdrawing life support. They suggest ways to manage withdrawal of life support appropriately, through understanding the limits of treatment, expertly using palliative measures, communicating clearly with patients and families, and carefully orchestrating controllable events with compassion.

Francis Lee builds upon the preceding paper in his discussion of withdrawing life support in a special context: that of futile care ("Postoperative Futile Care: Stopping the Train When the Family Says 'Keep Going'"). After pointing out the difficulties in the definition of futile care, he discusses the conflicts that may arise when a surgeon believes that further life support should be withdrawn because it is not medically indicated and the family disagrees; describes how to negotiate conflict by discovering and understanding the values that drive the family's viewpoint; and asserts the ultimate irrelevance of fears about lawsuits when making decisions in the context of conflict.

In his article "Ethical Issues in Patient Safety," Lucian Leape brings us up to date on the current status of a field he virtually created over 25 years ago—dealing with medical and surgical errors and injury to patients. He begins with the ethical imperative to prevent errors and injury insofar as it is practical, then describes the necessity to search for new methods to prevent recurrences when errors are made, the ethical and practical necessity to be honest and open in dealing with patients, and taking responsibility both as individual surgeons and as a profession for ensuring that our surgical colleagues practice competently.

The section on Bioethics in Health Care Policy begins with a discussion of one of the major problems with public policy in the nation: how to provide health care for uninsured patients. John Goodman applies the do-no-harm principle to this problem in his article "Solving the Problem of the Uninsured" by showing the harmful effects of some of the nation's health care policies and suggesting ways to fix the system by converting some of those harms into goods.

Virtually every aspect of hospital practice and office practice has been affected by the implementation of HIPAA regulations over the past few years. Peter Angelos, in his article "Compliance with HIPAA Regulations: Ethics and Excesses," describes the well-accepted ethical foundations upon which most of the regulations are based, and attempts to quell the anxiety that many surgeons feel about disclosing patients' private information, fearing transgression of legal requirements that may subject them to substantial penalties or lawsuits.

The first transplant of a kidney was accomplished in December 1954, between identical twins. Living donors now provide several organs other than kidneys for transplantation, such as lobes of livers and lungs. In their article "The Ethics of Living Donor Lung Transplantation," Wells and Barr describe the special ethical considerations that are engendered by the risks of these procedures, which can be substantially greater than those of kidney transplantation.

In his article "Conflicts in the Surgeon's Duties to the Patient and to Society," Neil Farber describes a wide range of conflicts surgeons face between their obligations to individual patients and their broader obligations to society. He provides a model of analysis that may help in creating guidelines, as well as a mechanism that surgeons can use in balancing competing values when making a decision under such conflicts.

Grant and Iserson analyze the impact on patients of gifts to surgeons from pharmaceutical and device manufacturers. In their article "Who's Buying Lunch? Are Gifts to Surgeons from Industry Bad for Patients?", they present a strong case based on a great deal of indirect evidence that patients are indeed harmed by gifts to physicians from industry. They suggest that banning such gifts would not completely resolve the ethical problem, and they suggest a different, more effective solution.

In the section on Biomedical Research Ethics, Franklin Miller looks at aspects of surgical research that are distinct from those of other kinds of biomedical research. In his article "Ethical Issues in Surgical Research," he discusses such issues as the fuzzy boundary between innovative surgical practice and surgical research, the special problem with control groups in surgical trials, and nettlesome issues of informed consent for surgical research.

Haavi Morreim discusses the differences between clinical trials of surgical devices and drugs in her article "Surgically Implanted Devices: Ethical Challenges in a Very Different Kind of Research." She uses the AbioCor, a totally implantable heart replacement device, to highlight the differences between device trials and drug trials, such as much smaller numbers of subjects, incremental innovation within device trials, and limited possibilities of double-blinding, randomization, and placebo controls. She demonstrates convincingly that research on devices is, indeed, "a very different kind of research."

In presenting this collection of articles, we hope to achieve several goals: to stimulate CT surgeons to think analytically about their decision-making processes; to show that ethical considerations inform and motivate us in virtually every aspect of our day-to-day professional activities; to demonstrate that ethical thought and deliberation have a crucial role to play in developing health care policy; and to highlight the special characteristics of clinical trials in surgery that make them in some ways unsuitable for the theoretically ideal methods of research that we learned in medical school. In striving for these goals, we hope in some small way to help surgeons to increase the first and decrease the second objective in the not-so-ancient aphorism "Above all, do more good than harm."

Robert M. Sade, MD
Department of Surgery
Institute of Human Values in Health Care
Medical University of South Carolina
96 Jonathan Lucas Street, Suite 409
P.O. Box 250612
Charleston, SC 29425, USA
E-mail address: sader@musc.edu

References

[1] Smith CM. Origin and uses of *primum non nocere*, above all, do no harm! J Clin Pharmacol 2005;45:371–7.
[2] Wikipedia. Primum non nocere. Available at: http://en.wikipedia.org/wiki/Primum_non_nocere. Accessed July 6, 2005.
[3] Council on Ethical and Judicial Affairs. Code of medical ethics, current opinions and annotations, 2004–2005. Chicago: American Medical Association; 2004.
[4] Paola F, Barton SS. An "ethics gap" in writing about bioethics: a quantitative comparison of the medical and surgical literature. J Med Ethics 1995;21:84–8.
[5] Sade RM, Williams T, Haney C, et al. The ethics gap in surgery. Ann Thorac Surg 2000;69:326–9.

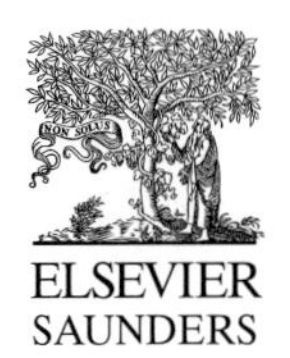
ELSEVIER
SAUNDERS

Thorac Surg Clin 15 (2005) 451 – 460

THORACIC
SURGERY
CLINICS

Informed Consent: It's Not Just Signing a Form

James W. Jones, MD, PhD[a,*], Lawrence B. McCullough, PhD[b], Bruce W. Richman, MA[c]

[a] *31 LaCosta Road, Montgomery, TX 77356, USA*
[b] *Center for Medical Ethics and Health Policy, Baylor College of Medicine, One Baylor Plaza, Houston, TX 77030, USA*
[c] *2809 Butterfield Court, Columbia, MO 65203, USA*

The clinical skills required in the informed consent process tend not to be taught to fellows, residents, and medical students within the formal curriculum [1]. Furthermore, surgical residents are seldom supervised during their communication with patients. As a result, faculty and trainees alike forego an opportunity to identify, evaluate, and address weaknesses in the resident's interpersonal skills with patients generally, and during the informed consent dialogue in particular. Surgical practice is distinct from nonsurgical medical practice in a number of regards, primarily because of the operation. Surgical therapy occurs as a specific event, usually requiring entry into the patient's body; the therapeutic event can be timed exactly (assigning culpability); the emotional stress on the patient is greater; and the surgical patient plays a more passive role than patients of other medical specialties once anesthesia is induced. The patient then becomes incapable of participatory intraoperative decision-making; and surgeon assumes full control of the decision-making process. Surgeons may consequently have a less fully developed sense of an active physician-patient partnership in the healing process than colleagues in other specialties, and this can affect their approach to informed consent. The surgeon may also assume that the referring physician has already made the necessary intellectual and emotional preparations and effectively has obtained the patient's consent for surgical resolution of the clinical problem. In combination, these factors can lead the unwitting surgeon to underestimate the capacity and willingness of the patient to participate in the informed consent process that should precede induction of anesthesia. As a consequence, the surgeon can lose the opportunity to form an effective therapeutic alliance with the patient.

The informed consent process

Historical development

The traditional debate over the requirement that physicians involve patients in therapeutic decisions was transformed by the ethical and legal analysis of several important legal cases involving surgical treatment. The starting point is the common law of informed consent as a patient's right, a twentieth century concept. Two key features of the legal history of informed consent are relevant here: simple consent and informed consent.

Simple consent involves one question: "Did the patient agree to be treated"? If the answer is yes, then the conditions of consent are thought to be satisfied. If the answer is no, then the conditions are not satisfied and the surgeon cannot operate.

In 1914, Judge Benjamin Cardozo wrote a landmark opinion in the case *Schloendorff v The Society of New York Hospital*, which legally defined simple consent and changed the history of American medical ethics [2]. Cardozo wrote that, "every human being of adult years and sound mind has a right to de-

* Corresponding author.
E-mail address: jwjones@bcm.tmc.edu (J.W. Jones).

1547-4127/05/$ – see front matter
doi:10.1016/j.thorsurg.2005.06.001

termine what shall be done with his body; and a surgeon who performs an operation without his patient's consent commits an assault, for which he is liable in damages, ... except in cases of emergency, where the patient is unconscious, and where it is necessary to operate before consent can be obtained" [2]. The patient's autonomy was at least equally important. Respect for autonomy obligates the physician to seek for the patient the greater balance of goods over harms, as those goods and harms are understood and balanced from the patient's perspective. The surgeon no longer possessed authority to act unilaterally on clinical judgments.

Although many surgeons today practice as though simple consent is still the ethical standard, the subsequent legal history of informed consent focused on the nature and quality of the physician's disclosure and obligation. Instead of one question, two questions must be asked: "Did the physician provide the patient with an adequate amount of information?", and "On the basis of this information, did the patient consent?" As the common law developed from the late 1950s through the early 1970s, two standards of adequacy emerged. The first is the professional community or professional practice standard [3,4]. Under this physician-oriented standard of disclosure, the patient should be told what an appropriately experienced physician in the community would tell the patient about the patient's condition, alternatives available for managing the condition, and generalize the benefits and risks of each alternative.

The courts gradually came to regard the professional community standard as inadequate, largely because of growing skepticism about the integrity of a solely physician-based standard. A major event in the development of an alternative standard was the case of *Canterbury v Spence*, decided in 1972 but occurring in 1958 [5]. This court rejected the professional community standard as inadequate and replaced it with the reasonable person standard. Informed consent involves meeting the needs of the "reasonable patient." This legal construct means that the informational needs of a patient should be identified on the basis of what a reasonable patient, not a particular patient in a particular, subjective circumstance, needs to know to make a meaningful decision. The patient needs to know material information (ie, what the nonprofessional patient is unlikely to encounter in daily life). The discussion need not be a disquisition, and surely the physician is not compelled to give his or her patient a short medical education; the disclosure role summons the physician only to a reasonable explanation. This means generally informing the patient in nontechnical terms what is at stake.

Patients may need, and often welcome, an offer to help think through their options. Because the decisions often involve subtle tradeoffs that are best understood and judged only by the patient, the surgeon should monitor himself or herself against coercing the patient, overtly or subtly. He or she may, and should, present the best case for surgical treatment if it is professionally considered to be the safest and most effective course, but the detriments of other alternatives or the benefits of surgery should not be exaggerated. In explaining the risks and discomforts attendant to any course, surgeons should be wary of making these sound so frightening that the patient rejects all varieties of crucial treatment.

In addition to the obligation to obtain consent or refusal, the patient's "yes" or "no" to intervention, the reasonable person standard includes a duty to explain clinical judgments and recommendations that enable the patient to make an independent, informed decision. The patient's perspective of his or her own interests should be respected by the surgeon. The ethical principle of respect for autonomy captures what is at stake clinically. The surgeon should acknowledge and accept the integrity of the competent patient's values and beliefs, whether or not the surgeon agrees with them, and should provide the patient with an adequate amount of information. A physician's disclosure is adequate when it includes the salient features of the physician's clinical thinking in arriving at the recommended therapy and explains to the patient the basic thought process that brought the surgeon to the conclusion that surgical management is a reasonable course of therapeutic action for this patient in this case [1].

The process

Surgeons should conceptualize and practice informed consent as a continuing process, rather than as a static event. Properly used, informed consent provides the basis for a strong and enduring professional alliance between the surgeon and patient, with shared responsibility for decision making [4]. Thus understood, informed consent is not simply the signature on the authorization form. This is legal documentation, and whereas documentation is important in satisfying the legal component of the consent process, documentation does not constitute the most important ethical element of informed consent. The patient's signature on the informed consent form is far less crucial than the process that it serves to document.

The concept of informed consent includes three elements, each of which presumes and builds on its predecessor [4]. The first is disclosure by the surgeon to the patient of adequate clear information about the patient's diagnosis; the alternatives available to treat the patient's problem, including surgical and nonsurgical management; the benefits and risks of each alternative, including nonintervention (ie, allowing the natural history of the disease to continue); and a frank explanation of those factors about which the medical profession, and the individual surgeon in particular, are uncertain and cannot provide guarantees. This disclosure should be individually tailored in its presentation to the intellectual and emotional capacity of each patient to understand, absorb, and retain information and make decisions. The second of the three elements is the patient's understanding of this clinical information. The third element is the patient's process of decision, based not only on what the surgeon has told them, but information they have been exposed to from other sources, including other physicians, family and friends, and perhaps an acquaintance who has had a similar procedure; what they have read by independently researching the problem; and their own emotional response to illness and all that it changes in one's life. The ethical requirements of each of these three elements are now considered in greater clinical detail.

Disclosure obligations

No surgeon wants to be sued, lose patients' confidence, or undergo the humiliation of admitting errors; all are among the distinct dangers of full disclosure. The spirit of informed consent, however, has ethically and legally replaced paternalism in surgery. Informed consent does not stop with the agreement to accept therapy [6]. Mutual decision-making by the physician and patient (or family, when the patient agrees or cannot participate) about treatment has the same ethical obligations throughout the course of therapy.

Kantian ethics suggest that although one must avoid deception, truth may be selectively told. Selective truth telling is the way personal lives are lived; one chooses to whom one discloses information or not, and the sensitivity or completeness of information disclosed. This ethical axiom does not apply in the surgeon-patient relationship concerning specifics of the patient's condition and therapy. The physician must help the patient to understand both what is planned preoperatively and how treatment is proceeding. The extent of disclosure is generally based on the physician's identification of information that should influence diagnosis, treatment planning, and outcomes. This includes knowledge that the average layperson cannot be expected to have, but needs to know to participate meaningfully in treatment decisions and planning for the future.

The patient's understanding

McKneally and Martin [7] examined the consent process before major surgery from the patient's perspective. Several recurrent themes of patient's mental processes were learned: a belief in surgical cure, enhancement of trust through the referral process, idealization of the specialist surgeon, belief in expertise rather than medical information, resignation to risks of treatment, and acceptance of an expert recommendation as consent to treatment. Those patients with serious illnesses, being sent to a specific surgeon or a specific institution, had already firmly committed to operative therapy and the consent process was a formality. Patients constructed their belief systems through faith before the informed consent process took place. Informed consent in surgical practice must respond to these ethical challenges and opportunities. The surgeon should consider informed consent as an ethically essential course of action that can be used to strengthen the surgeon-patient alliance with mutual benefits. Although surgeons hesitate to mention it and its real effect is unquantified, there is a noteworthy placebo effect in surgery [8] that should not be overlooked.

Apart from legal considerations that are minimal by professional moral standards, surgeons must always remember that having major surgery is one of the most stressful and fearful events of patients' lives. The law emphasizes the physician's role in the informed consent process. This is not surprising; patients bring tort actions against the physicians, not vice versa. The courts have not been asked to address the patient's role in the informed consent process. Ethics addresses both the physician's and the patient's roles and responsibilities in the informed consent transaction. Ethical consideration goes on to evaluate what the surgeon has explained and what the patient has understood, the second substantive element in informed consent. Patients need to understand what surgeons tell them about a proposed surgical procedure.

More substantively, patients need to understand that they are being asked to authorize surgical management. Faden and Beauchamp [4] point out that this means that the patient must understand that by consenting to surgical management the patient authorizes the surgeon and surgical team to perform the procedure that the surgeon has described to the patient. The patient must also understand that the surgery cannot proceed without the patient's permission.

Finally, the patient should understand what is being authorized [4,9]. The patient needs to grasp the nature of the procedure, its goals, its expected duration, and what can be expected during the near- and long-term recovery process. Sequelae of surgery, particularly functional changes that affect job performance, valued activities, or sexuality, and aesthetic changes, such as the length and appearance of scar tissue, must be understood.

Documentation in the medical record

A well-crafted note in the medical record can be a valuable clinical aid to the surgeon, as a checklist and record of the information exchanged. The consent note should include a listing of the people in attendance, the description of the procedure in lay terms, the goal of the procedure as described (with any figures about failure rates), the major aspects or steps of the procedure that were discussed, the benefits and risks of the procedure which were discussed and the pertinent questions asked, as well as expectations for the course of both near- and long-term recovery. The note should specify that the patient authorizes the surgeon and surgical team to perform the procedure. The contents of the note can be reviewed with the patient and the patient encouraged to identify what is still unclear or confusing, so that these matters can be addressed.

The process of deciding

Patient's psychology during consent

McKneally and Martin [7] found that many patients have already determined the absolute necessity of surgical therapy before seeing the surgeon and are focused on obtaining operations; the informed consent process should both supply the necessary information and serve to qualify the patient's belief system.

The process of making an explicit decision by the patient on the surgeon's recommendation is importantly placed as the third and culminating element of the informed consent process. In making their decisions about surgery, patients should appreciate that present conditions and actions have future consequences. The patient should be able to reason from present events to future consequences and have an adequately developed sense of the probabilities that these projected outcomes, called cognitive understanding, may indeed occur. The surgeon's important role in the development of cognitive understanding includes correcting errors in the patient's information, helping to augment the patient's fund of knowledge, and helping patients grasp the nature and likelihood of the future consequences attendant on each of the therapeutic choices available to them.

In response to patients who desire only a small role in the decision-making process but want surgical management of their problem, the surgeon should nonetheless provide an explanation of the surgical procedure by reviewing the major issues, such as contents of the consent form. The surgeon should also prepare the patient for the immediate postoperative period with a brief explanation of what this entails so that the patient is not surprised or alarmed when they wake up in the recovery area or surgical intensive care unit.

Patients considering surgery should also evaluate benefits and risks of the alternatives available to them. These are value judgments and concern how much worth to attach to potential favorable and unfavorable outcomes associated with each available option. Making such value judgments involves evaluative understanding, a clinical consideration overlooked altogether in the law governing informed consent. In making decisions about surgery, each patient needs to make value judgments about the benefits, risks, and discomforts of surgery; of other available medical interventions; and whether surgery or other invention is less dire than living with the risks and discomforts of untreated illness. Evaluative understanding is just as essential to the patient's decision-making as cognitive understanding.

The surgeon can help the patient to develop evaluative understanding of available alternatives. Asking a patient, "What is important to you as you consider . . .," with the ellipsis completed with each alternative, is effective in eliciting the patient's values [10]. The surgeon should discern patterns of values in conversation with the patient and identify them for patients who are struggling to articulate what is important to them. Patients do not make decisions on the basis of isolated values, and helping patients to connect otherwise unarticulated concerns promotes individual autonomy. They might consider job performance, sexual activity, mental function, physical appearance, and, particularly important, hobbies of the retired to define their values. For example, it does not respect the values of a patient who is an avid hunter to place a pacemaker on the side of the chest from which the patient fires a shotgun while dove hunting. Such assistance also directs the surgeon's relationship to the patient's most fundamental values and beliefs because they give meaning to the alternative possible futures the patient must contemplate. Evaluative understanding is the area that may depart most radically from the surgeon's own value system, requiring a nondirective approach. Once the patient has identified his or her relevant values and evaluated the alternatives on this basis, it is time for the surgeon to offer a recommendation.

The patient should not only feel free to ask questions, but should be encouraged to do so. The meaning of questions from the patient and the patient's family is not always readily apparent. The first question of many patients is often, "How long will this operation take?", and the surgeon should respond with an estimate of the customary range of time it has taken them to complete this procedure in the past. The surgeon should also understand that the real question being asked usually is, "When should my family begin to worry that things aren't going well?". To help patients with questions they have difficulty articulating, the surgeon may direct the conversation to questions that earlier patients have asked about this procedure, and invite the patient to discuss these questions in the context of their personal concerns. Patients usually become relaxed enough to start asking their own questions and genuinely begin to seek information about the operation.

Respect for the autonomy of the patient means that the patient's decision should be free of substantially controlling influences [4,11]. The physician should make a recommendation only after the patient has developed evaluative understanding without fear of bringing undue influence to bear on the patient's autonomy. Most patients highly value the surgeon's recommendation as they struggle to reach their own decisions. Appropriately timed recommendations play an important role in the informed consent process, and may even support the independent nature of the patient's decision.

The ethics of the informed consent process emphasizes the role of this process in developing solid rapport with the patient. Such a rapport has a number of clinical advantages. First, the surgeon does not function as a disinterested and unbiased source of information, consulted as one might consult a book as a noninteractive source. Instead, the surgeon has important experiences and opinions with which to assist the patient in the decision-making process, not the least important of which are the technical information and knowledge of the patient's personal medical history. Failure by surgeons to provide patients with the full range of their knowledge for fear of violating a patient's autonomy could mean that the patient does not become genuinely informed, and ultimately defeats the high-minded principle the surgeon is seeking to protect the patient. Ultimately, no one knows more or is more intimately concerned about the details of the patient's surgical treatment than the surgeon and the patient, which makes their mutually respectful cooperation essential to the process of genuine informed consent. Second, forming a therapeutic alliance with the patient through the informed consent process results in a more informed, prepared patient, who has developed a sense of individual responsibility in the transaction. Patient compliance may increase, leading to a smoother, more effective postoperative course. In an era of managed care, this outcome helps to promote the valued goal of the more economically efficient use of expensive medical resources, like surgery. Third, the open and honest two-way communication called for by the ethics of the informed consent process should increase the patient's confidence and trust in the surgeon. This goes a long way toward establishing good rapport with patients, and advance the value of surgery for both surgeon and patient.

Definition of the process

Formed by this ethical analysis, the informed consent process becomes a process of mutual decision-making. The surgeon and the patient both have active and important roles in this process, and responsibilities to discharge. The surgeon, as the patient's fiduciary, should share beneficence-based clinical judgment with the patient. As the patient's fiduciary (ie, as someone who acts primarily to protect the patient's interests), the surgeon should also be committed to doing the right thing for the patient, but the ultimate decision about what is right for the patient rests with the patient. For this reason, the ethics of the informed consent process places strong emphasis on the surgeon's respect for the patient's autonomy.

Initiation of the consent process in the surgical holding area just before the operation is scheduled to begin should be avoided in all but the most urgent or most minor procedures. Instead, the discussion should be initiated well in advance of surgery because decisions should be made without added tension and with the time necessary to a major life decision. Outpatient visits for preoperative work-up provide an ideal opportunity to conduct the informed consent process.

Extent of the surgeon's influence

The surgeon's recommendations have a proper role in the informed consent process. Most patients value their surgeon's recommendations and customarily give them considerable weight in their own decision-making process about whether to accept surgical management of their condition. In principle, surgeons exercise permissible influence through their recommendations.

Altering the frame of reference to influence the patient's decision by excessively emphasizing either benefits or risks, a process termed "framing" [1], poses clinical ethical challenges. Framing is inconsistent with both the surgeon's fiduciary role and with respect for patient autonomy, and should be avoided. For example, the surgeon may describe surgical risks as merely routine, as they may seem to the surgeon, and the benefits as certain. These descriptions may be consistent with the individual surgeon's experience, but they are incorrect in terms of predicting the outcome for the specific operative patient and are deceptive. Inadvertently, a surgeon may seek to reassure a patient by making such statements as "I cannot remember the last time we lost a patient from this operation." Framing in this manner before the patient decides to have surgery is ethically questionable, because the characterization can discourage development of the patient's own critical evaluation.

Surgeons should also avoid a particularly corrupt and common type of framing commonly termed "crepe hanging." This involves exaggerating the gravity of the patient's situation, and of the operation, to increase the patient's estimation of and gratitude toward the surgeon when things go well, as they were expected to by the surgeon in the first place. Should the surgery have a poor outcome, the surgeon has only to say that this is as he predicted and the patient nevertheless agreed to proceed.

Surgeons should be especially aware of subtle framing effects that can occur when substituting descriptive terms for quantitative terms, especially in the characterization of risks. For example, the surgeon might tell the patient facing surgery for glaucoma, "You will lose your eyesight without the procedure." The more truthful statement, however, is that a certain percentage of people in this circumstance, perhaps 15% in this hypothetical case, lose eyesight without the corrective procedure. Surgeons should adhere to quantitative descriptions whenever possible in the early steps of the informed consent process and then help the patient to evaluate this information in the steps concerned with cognitive and evaluative understanding.

Special circumstances during informed consent

Conflicting professional opinions

Patients occasionally encounter conflicting opinions among surgeons or between the referring physician and the referral surgeon. Everyone in the medical profession understands, but may not readily acknowledge, that clinical judgment can vary widely among the specialties and even among practitioners within the same specialty. For example, the referring physician may focus on the operation's morbidity risks, whereas the surgeon may be most concerned about reducing disease-related mortality and so may discount, to some extent, the inconvenience, cost, morbidity, and discomfort of the procedure [12]. The guiding principle when differences of judgment occur was articulated two centuries ago by the Scottish physician John Gregory (1724–1773). He emphasized that the surgeons and physicians should manage such disagreements with a view always toward protecting the interests of the patient [12].

Consent with multiple physicians

The typical surgical patient receives ongoing care from physicians in several specialties, including surgery, before, during, and after procedures. The tendency exists in these team contexts to assume that others have already spoken with the patient, have explained what is happening, and have taken the patient through the informed consent process. This assumption can lead to a defective informed consent process, especially regarding the surgical procedure being contemplated. The operating surgeon should take a preventive ethics approach to this potential problem by accepting responsibility for taking the patient through the consent process for the operation. The anesthesiologist should participate in this process with reference to the alternatives, benefits, and effects of anesthesia options. All physicians, especially those in training, should avoid giving answers to questions outside their specialty and about which they are uncertain, and avoid areas apart from their expertise.

When multiple surgeons are involved, the surgical specialist who performs the most essential and most complication-prone parts of the operation has the greatest responsibility regarding informed consent. This physician should tell the patient who the other participants are and what their roles will be in the patient's care. This preventive ethics approach minimizes the chance that the patient will become confused or concerned about the involvement of multiple surgeons.

Patients who are undecided or refuse surgery

Some patients may refuse surgical intervention after an adequate informed consent process because they are in a state of indecision. If the consent process has gone well, this indecision usually results from a patient's ambivalence over similarly attractive alternatives. The patient may often also be frightened about having an operation and understandably may resolve indecision in favor of nonsurgical management of the condition.

In this case the surgeon should explain that the patient has caused no offense by being undecided. Such a decision, after all, does not preclude a decision for surgery later. In elective surgeries, the patient should be encouraged to think matters through and to determine if the decision will become more apparent with time. The surgeon should explain, however, that the postponement of surgical treatment, as cases of cancers, for example, may change the nature of benefits and risks. If the surgeon decides to remain on such a patient's case, the patient should be so informed, and told that the surgeon will discuss the patient's decision at any time. The canons of medical ethics and common courtesy are violated if the surgeon vocalizes disappointment, anger, or threatens to refuse future treatment toward the patient for not affirming trust in the consulting surgeon.

A patient's refusal to have surgery is not itself evidence of the patient's diminished decision-making capacity. Nonetheless, refusal when surgery is clearly indicated does raise a "red flag" and prompts any thoughtful surgeon to question the patient's decision-making capacity, especially in potentially life-threatening circumstances. A patient who refuses such surgery without attaching importance to mortality, morbidity, or reduced quality of life causes a surgeon frustration and concern. Recent studies of noncompliance confirm that failure in communication can result in patient refusal of the physician's recommendation, or noncooperation with a treatment plan [13].

The surgeon's first response to refusal of surgery should be to review with the patient his or her understanding of the condition, the nature of the surgical procedure, and its benefits and risks. The patient's cognitive understanding may be incomplete, and the patient may reconsider when more complete understanding has been developed. The surgeon's second response should be to explore the patient's evaluative understanding. Of particular concern should be possible mistrust of physicians (perhaps based on some prior experience); pressing obligations; or emotional factors like anxiety, depression, or fear. The surgeon's third response should be to acknowledge value conflicts when they occur, and work with the patient to identify a management plan that accords with the patient's values. If the surgeon believes that the patient's values are supported by surgery, the surgeon should point this out and ask the patient to reconsider. The preventive ethics approach to refusal of surgery should be respectful exploration of the patient's reasoning, on the assumption that patients, by their own lights, have good reasons for refusal but may, with additional information and reflection, reconsider and accept surgery. Surgeons should not assume that the patient's competence is somehow diminished or compromised just because he withholds consent.

One very helpful response to refusals when surgery's value in averting mortality is unclear is to offer the patient the alternative of a trial of nonsurgical management. Nonsurgical management may be supported by patient values that emerge during the consent process. The patient should be informed of this possibility and a mutual plan developed to monitor the nonsurgical trial of management. The goal should be to identify mutually acceptable criteria for evaluating the nonsurgical management and for reconsidering it. Should a patient be disinclined to accept surgery or any other invasive management as the first option, the surgeon could propose a trial of medical management and agree with the patient on the conditions under which the surgeon initiates surgical intervention. Such circumstances could include recurrent and worsening pathology, even on a regular schedule of medication, unacceptable side effects of medication, or increasing risk of mortality.

Problems with the patient's decision-making capacity

Some patients may still experience difficulty making decisions, regardless of how ethically, astutely, and carefully the surgeon has attended to the informed consent process. The hospital's consultation-liaison psychiatrist, a physician who has the expertise to evaluate patients' decision-making capacity, can be a valuable advisor and ally. The patient should be told of the role of the psychiatrist to the extent that this is possible. The surgeon should make the following request. First, the psychiatrist should evaluate the patient for a formal cognitive or objective disorder or other psychiatric disturbance that might significantly affect the patient's ability to make decisions, and then determine whether the condition is susceptible to treatment. Second, the psychiatrist and the surgeon should agree on a clear delineation of boundaries in their treatment of the patient. Each should understand what the other will do to restore the patient's decision-making capacity and cooperate with one another. Third, the psychiatrist and surgeon should develop a plan for improving the patient's decision-making capacity so that the patient is able to participate in the informed consent process. In all cases, the surgeon should not use consultation-liaison psychiatry simply to declare a patient incompetent [13], thereby enabling others to make decisions for the patient, or discharging the patient to the management of other specialties. Patients with waxing and waning decisional capacity often experience periods of lucidity, and may choose to provide informed consent for surgery during such a period, specifying that statements they may subsequently make while confused should not supersede decisions made during a period of lucidity. These have been called "Ulysses contracts" in the bioethics literature [1,14].

Surrogate decisions

Working up the patient who exhibits problems with decision-making capacity with the aid of consultation-liaison psychiatry should lead to the reliable identification of patients who have irreversibly lost the capacity to participate in the decision-making process. By common law and now in many states by statutory law, family members are asked to make decisions for such patients [15]. There is a stable consensus in the bioethics literature for how this process should occur [14].

Family members should not be asked, "What would you do?" or "What do you want to do?", because these questions invite family members inadvertently to mix up their own concerns and values with those of the patient. Family members should be asked what they believe is important to the patient at this time and in these circumstances. The goal is to try to construct what the patient's evaluative understanding is as closely as possible. On this basis, the remaining steps of the consent process should be completed. This leads to what is known as "substituted judgment" [14].

Sometimes, for a variety of reasons, family members cannot achieve substituted judgment. In such cases they should be asked to make the decision that in their view protects and promotes their loved one's interests. The best way to assist family members in these circumstances is to encourage patients to take a preventive ethics approach on their own. All patients in their geriatric years, those with chronic diseases, and those in the early stages of dementia should be encouraged to express their values and preferences in advance. Advance directives have legal standing in most states.

Surrogate decisions that inaccurately represent the patient's wishes are not ethically binding on the surgeon, provided the surgeon has a basis for reasonable certainty that the surrogate is mistaken before acting contrary to the surrogate's instructions [14]. When the disputed decision is important enough, the court can be petitioned for appointment of a conservator. Surrogate decision-making fails to reflect the patient's wishes accurately in 70% of important treatment issues [16]. If the surgeon chooses to override the faulty surrogate decision when the surrogate is otherwise entitled to control an important decision, surgeon-family conflicts are likely. It is wise to notify the institutional ethics committee or chief of staff in such cases.

Pediatric consent

As a matter of law, parents are in authority over their minor children and are empowered to engage in the informed consent process on their child's behalf. Minor children, however, are not mere objects; they have their own values and preferences for how they want to receive health care. The American Academy of Pediatrics supports the view that children should participate in decision-making commensurate with their developmental capacity [17]. Pediatric surgeons confront conceptual and clinical challenges regarding pediatric assent. Adolescent patients, particularly those with chronic diseases about which the patient has become quite knowledgeable and mature, may be able to complete the steps of the informed consent process as well as adults. When this is the case, the patient's autonomy should be respected by the surgeon and by the adolescent's parents. In these circumstances the surgeon's responsibilities include pointing out to the parents that their child is capable of making an adult decision that deserves respect. When there are differences between parent and child, the surgeon should offer his or her services as a good-faith negotiator. The goal should be to reach a commonly accepted decision rather than to decide whose decision wins.

Not all adolescents can complete the informed consent process, nor can younger children. Nonetheless, children are capable of understanding to a degree appropriate to their age and emotional development that they have a disease, what parts of the body the disease involves, and that surgery can help. These matters should be explained to the patient, when the goal is not so much to obtain the patient's consent as to provide information about the clinical course to which the patient's parents have already consented. This concept has led to such practices as familiarizing children with the hospital, including operative and postoperative areas, before elective surgery.

When supervised trainees do the surgery

The medical profession has an ethical and social obligation to educate physicians and surgeons to meet the needs of future generations of patients. The first teaching hospitals in America were modeled on the British infirmaries and funded from public and private sources. These hospitals provided free care to the poor, and were seen by academic physicians as training sites where a presumed sense of reciprocity obligates indigent patients to serve willingly as teaching material in exchange for their care [18]. This assumption is now considered incompatible with the process of informed consent, which is understood to include the patient's awareness and agreement that trainees may participate in the treatment process. The American Medical Association Council on Ethical and Judicial Affairs has established a clear position on the relationship between patients and trainees on clinical rotations: "Patients should be informed of the identity and training status of individuals involved in their care, and all health care professionals share the responsibility for properly identifying themselves" [19]. Before patients can accept the role of teaching subject, they must be made aware that they have been offered the part.

Informed consent in research

Some ethical constructs, particularly those involving informed consent and the conduct of research, have been so uniformly accepted as necessary to the rights of patients and the integrity of scientific method that they have been codified into international declarations and federal law. Sade [20] summarized the various historical proclamations and their ethical implications in scientific publication. Once surgery embarks into research, surgical autonomy has compelling ethical limits. When the selection process for a medication, graft, or implant is randomized or preassigned, when the choice is not primarily determined or influenced by the patient's individual clinical characteristics, or when the clinical outcome cannot be predicted and alternatives exist, the procedure must be considered clinical research rather than clinical care, and the laws, customs, restrictions, and ethical considerations specific to research become applicable. Surgeons must modify their own behavior accordingly, and observe the legal and ethical conventions that ensure integrity of scientific investigation and the safety of research subjects. Institutional approval must be sought and received before initiation of a research study to ensure the soundness of the science and the safety of patients.

References

[1] McCullough L, Jones JW, Brody BA. Informed consent: autonomous decision making of the surgical patient. In: McCullough LB, Jones JW, Brody BA, editors. Surgical ethics. New York: Oxford University Press; 1998.
[2] *Schloendorff v Society of New York Hospital*, 211 NY 125, 126, 105 NE 92, (1914).
[3] Wear S. Enhancing clinician provision of informed consent and counseling: some pedagogical strategies. J Med Philos 1999;24:34–42.
[4] Faden R, Beachamp T. A history and theory of informed consent. New York: Oxford University Press; 1986.
[5] *Canterbury v Spense*, 464 F2d 772, 785 (DC Cir 1972).
[6] Jones JW, McCullough LB. Disclosure of intraoperative events. Surgery 2002;132:531–2.
[7] McKneally MF, Martin DK. An entrustment model of consent for surgical treatment of life-threatening illness: perspective of patients requiring esophagectomy. J Thorac Cardiovasc Surg 2000;120:264–9.
[8] Moseley JB, O'Malley K, Petersen NJ, et al. A controlled trial of arthroscopic surgery for osteoarthritis of the knee. N Engl J Med 2002;347:81–8.
[9] Wear S. Informed consent: patient autonomy and physician beneficence with clinical medicine. Dordrecht: Kluwer Academic Publishers; 1993.
[10] McCullough L, Wilson B, Teasdale NL, et al. Mapping personal, familial, and professional values in long-term care decisions. Gerontologist 1993;33:324–32.
[11] Jones JW, McCullough LB. Refusal of life-saving treatment in the aged. J Vasc Surg 2002;35:1067.
[12] Jones JW, McCullough LB, Richman BW. Management of disagreements between attending and consulting physicians. J Vasc Surg 2003;38:1137–8.
[13] Jones JW, McCullough LB, Richman BW. The surgeon's obligations to the noncompliant patient. J Vasc Surg 2003;38:626–7.
[14] Buchanan A, Brock D. Deciding for others: the ethics of surrogate decision making. New York: Cambridge University Press; 1989.
[15] Areen J. The legal status of consent obtained from families of adult patients to withhold or withdraw treatment. JAMA 1987;258:229–35.
[16] Hare J, Pratt C, Nelson C. Agreement between patients

and their self-selected surrogates on difficult medical decisions. Arch Intern Med 1992;152:1049–54.
[17] Committee on Bioethics, American Academy of Pediatrics. Informed consent, parental permission, and assent in pediatric practice. Pediatrics 1995;95:314–7.
[18] Bard S. A discourse upon the duties of a physician. In: Bard S, editor. Two discourses dealing with medical education in early New York. New York: Columbia University Press; 1921.
[19] Jones JW, McCullough LB. Consent for residents to perform surgery. J Vasc Surg 2002;36:655–6.
[20] Sade RM. Publication of unethical research studies: the importance of informed consent. Ann Thorac Surg 2003;75:325–8.

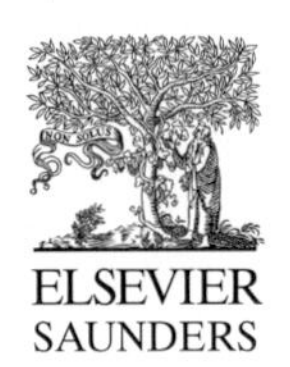
ELSEVIER
SAUNDERS

Thorac Surg Clin 15 (2005) 461 – 468

THORACIC
SURGERY
CLINICS

The Effect of Patients' Noncompliance on Their Surgeons' Obligations

Jay A. Jacobson, MD, FACP

Division of Medical Ethics, Department of Internal Medicine, LDS Hospital and University of Utah School of Medicine, Salt Lake City, UT 84143, USA

I recently had an instructive encounter with the word, "obligation." Senior medical students had met, heard, and interacted with Paul Farmer, the Tanner Lecturer on human values. Dr. Farmer is an internationally respected physician who has dedicated his life and work to treatment of people in the developing world. More students than could be accommodated responded when invited to have lunch with Dr. Farmer. They eagerly queried him about opportunities to work with underserved populations. The next week in the Medical Ethics course, I asked all 104 students if they believed they had any obligation to serve the world's poorest and most vulnerable populations. I was stunned when no one raised a hand. I acknowledged my surprise and asked them to share their reaction to the question. Many of them expressed interest, willingness, desire, and even a plan to do some medical service in the Third World. All of them, however, took issue with the concept of obligation. They were looking forward to their medical independence and freedom from the regimentation of medical school and the constraints of residency. Maybe it was the added awareness of their enormous loans, but "obligation" triggered strong negative reactions. They recognized that they were obliged to complete residencies to practice medicine, but they did not recognize a universal obligation to serve any particular patient or patient population. They resented the idea that others expected or asserted such a duty.

These soon-to-be physicians were young and inexperienced. They had not yet sworn any oaths, received their licenses, or signed any contracts. Nevertheless, their reactions and comments made me realize that I may have made some assumptions about physicians' obligations to patients that were not widely shared and perhaps not well supported. They reminded me that physicians value their freedom, autonomy, and authority, and do not welcome the idea of being told what to do or being obliged to do it. The students also reminded me that people prefer and enjoy work they want to do more than work they have to do.

Few prefer or enjoy working with "noncompliant" patients, but this article explores whether clinicians, surgeons in particular, are obliged to take care of them. The sources for professional and personal obligations to patients are considered; there are some obligations, but they are specific and contextual. Also examined are what actions exempt surgeons from these obligations and whether noncompliance per se always or sometimes constitutes such an exemption. Because there is an obligation to treat at least some noncompliant patients, ways to identify those patients and strategies to make working with them more effective and less onerous are suggested.

What are surgeons' professional and personal obligations to patients?

Many look to the Hippocratic Oath as a statement of medicine's principles and priorities [1]. It might

E-mail address: ldjacob@ihc.com

1547-4127/05/$ – see front matter
doi:10.1016/j.thorsurg.2005.06.012

thoracic.theclinics.com

clarify professional obligations. It pledges that clinicians will act for the benefit of the patient, but it does not explain how someone gets to be the patient. Once someone becomes the patient, the oath obliges one to respect his or her confidence and not reveal embarrassing information. The oath obliges one not to prescribe a deadly drug or to participate in birth control. It is silent about whether noncompliance relieves one of any obligation. The oath may not even be relevant or applicable to surgeons because it was intended for other kinds of physicians, as reflected in the statement: "I will not use the knife, not even on sufferers from stone, but will withdraw in favor of such men as are engaged in this work" [1]. The oath, ostensibly written in the fourth century BC and probably by someone other than Hippocrates, seems more than a bit dated now and does not reflect changes in medical knowledge, technology, ethics, and law. It would not be regarded as binding unless one swore to it and even then there is no real mechanism for monitoring adherence or sanctions based on a breach of this promise.

Most physicians actually take quite a different oath when they complete medical school. Today, the "Oath of Lasagna" is one of several oaths that have been offered to replace the original Hippocratic Oath while preserving its spirit [2]. Other alternatives include the Oath of Maimonides, attributed to the twelfth-century Jewish physician Moses Maimonides [3], and the Declaration of Geneva [4], composed by the World Medical Association in 1948. The latter is, in part, reactive and responsive to the terrible, involuntary medical experiments conducted by German physicians in World War II. The trend among many medical schools is to have each graduating class hammer out an oath of its own that reflects the professional ideals of its members [5]. Although these newer oaths add new obligations, such as securing voluntary, informed consent for research, they make no mention of an obligation to treat all patients. They do not mention noncompliance.

Interestingly, the earliest American Medical Association's (AMA) Code of Ethics in 1847 included what could be regarded as a code of expected behavior for patients [6]. "The obedience of a patient to the prescriptions of his physician should be prompt and implicit. He should never permit his own crude opinions as to their fitness, to influence his attention to them...This remark is equally applicable to diet, drink, and exercise." It urged patients to be compliant with medical instructions. That code also omitted any generic obligation to care for all or a particular class of patients, but it did mention obligations to patients in one's practice. It did not indicate whether patient noncompliance could excuse doctors from these obligations.

The current AMA Code of Ethics reflects the larger changes in American society that have diminished the unquestioned authority of leaders and professionals and elevated the autonomy and rights of individuals and classes of persons, including patients [7]. The long tradition of medical paternalism, doctor knows best, and following doctor's "orders" is no longer widely accepted by the American public or supported by laws related to patient decision making. The AMA Code now has a brief section that includes patient responsibilities. Its language reflects an incomplete transition between an earlier era of doctor-directed care and a currently envisioned negotiated partnership between doctor and patient.

> It has long been recognized that successful medical care requires an ongoing collaborative effort between patients and physicians. Physician and patient are bound in a partnership that requires both individuals to take an active role in the healing process. Such a partnership does not imply that both partners have identical responsibilities or equal power. While physicians have the responsibility to provide health care services to patients to the best of their ability, patients have the responsibility to communicate openly, to participate in decisions about the diagnostic and treatment recommendations, and to comply with the agreed-upon treatment program. Like patients' rights, patients' responsibilities are derived from the principle of autonomy. The principle of patient autonomy holds that an individual's physical, emotional, and psychological integrity should be respected and upheld. This principle also recognizes the human capacity to self-govern and choose a course of action from among different alternative options. Autonomous, competent patients assert some control over the decisions which direct their health care.
>
> ...Once patients and physicians agree upon the goals of therapy and a treatment plan, patients have a responsibility to cooperate with that treatment plan and to keep their agreed-upon appointments. Compliance with physician instructions is often essential to public and individual safety. Patients also have a responsibility to disclose whether previously agreed upon treatments are being followed and to indicate when they would like to reconsider the treatment plan.

Although not stating a universal professional obligation to care for all patients who request it, the current Code, which begins with nine principles, states in number 6: "A physician shall, in the provision of appropriate patient care, except in emergencies, be free to choose whom to serve, with whom to associate, and the environment in which to provide medical care" [8]. This suggests that there is an obligation to care for emergently ill patients. With respect to potential patients it seems that although there is a strong presumption that supports the physician's prerogative to choose whether to initiate a patient-physician relationship it can be superseded by an obligation to treat in specific circumstances. "Physicians cannot refuse to care for patients based on race, gender, sexual orientation, or any other criteria that would constitute invidious discrimination nor can they discriminate against patients with infectious diseases. Physicians may not refuse to care for patients when operating under a contractual arrangement that requires them to treat" [9].

Noncompliance does not excuse physicians from this specific obligation to accept potential patients, nor is it recognized to excuse them from principle 7, which applies to an established patient: "A physician shall, while caring for a patient, regard responsibility to the patient as paramount" [8]. Absent some specific obligation, such as those mentioned previously, however, the code states that physicians have the option of withdrawing from a case without mention of reasons. They should not neglect the patient, however, and they should not do so suddenly. "Physicians have an obligation to support continuity of care for their patients. While physicians have the option of withdrawing from a case, they cannot do so without giving notice to the patient, the relatives, or responsible friends sufficiently long in advance of withdrawal to permit another medical attendant to be secured" [10].

The AMA Code is cited frequently in legal cases related to professional conduct and violations of it could result in loss of AMA membership. Not all physicians and certainly not all surgeons belong to the AMA, however, and those who do not belong could claim that obligations in the Code do not apply to them. The code is also used by many state licensing boards as a behavioral standard for physicians regardless of AMA membership. A state board may sanction or revoke the license of a physician whose actions violate the code. It is difficult to identify self-imposed professional obligations of doctors without recourse to some type of code. The alternative is to refer to tradition or to turn to external sources, such as public expectation or the law.

Surgeons can refer to a variety of codes generally associated with specialties. Because the American College of Surgeons (ACS) has recently done extensive work on its code it is helpful to explore that code's statements about obligations to patients and the response to noncompliance.

The preamble of the ACS Code of Professional Conduct echoes the antidiscrimination language of the AMA Code, which reflects changes in civil rights and federal law, but it asserts a positive obligation to treat patients with respect and tolerance. The latter does seem relevant to the issue of noncompliance. "The ethical practice of medicine establishes and ensures an environment in which all individuals are treated with respect and tolerance; discrimination or harassment on the basis of age, sexual preference, gender, race, disease, disability, or religion, are proscribed as being inconsistent with the ideals and principles of the American College of Surgeons" [11].

The ACS Code itself, although it does not use the word "obligations," uses the word "responsibilities" and provides a short and incisive list of these with respect to "our patients." The most relevant ones are listed next [12]: "During the continuum of pre-, intra-, and postoperative care we accept responsibilities to:

- Serve as effective advocates for our patients' needs.
- Disclose therapeutic options, including their risks and benefits.
- Be sensitive and respectful of patients, understanding their vulnerability during the perioperative period.
- Acknowledge patients' psychological, social, cultural and spiritual needs."

In the section on competencies of the responsible surgeon five points seem directly related to noncompliance [13]. "A responsible surgeon should demonstrate competence in:

1. Patient Care that is compassionate, appropriate, and effective for the treatment of health problems and the promotion of good health.
2. Medical Knowledge about established and evolving biomedical, clinical, and cognate (for example, epidemiological and social-behavioral) sciences and the application of this knowledge to patient care.
3. Practice-Based Learning and Improvement that involves investigation and evaluation of a surgeon's patient care, appraisal and assimilation of scientific evidence, and improvements in patient care.
4. Interpersonal and Communication Skills that result in effective information exchange and effective interaction with patients, their families, and other health care professionals.
5. Professionalism, as manifested through a commitment to carrying out professional responsi-

bilities, adherence to ethical principles, and sensitivity to a diverse patient population."

In its section on the relation of the surgeon to the patient, the ACS code describes informed consent in terms of the proposed operation, but does not say anything about disclosing or agreeing on what medicines or treatments are required or recommended after it or what behaviors are inconsistent with optimal recovery and outcome. It does say, "When patients agree to an operation conditionally or make demands that are unacceptable to the surgeon; the surgeon may elect to withdraw from the case" [14]. This suggests that if a patient is informed about postoperative recommendations and requirements before an operation and refuses to comply with them, this could be regarded as an informed refusal to proceed or an ethical basis for the surgeon to withdraw or at least not to proceed with that particular treatment strategy. An alternative approach might be mutually acceptable to patient and surgeon.

It seems that although physicians are generally free to choose their patients, a person's emergent condition creates a duty to treat. Discrimination toward several identified classes or one's own contractual obligation precludes refusal to treat. Surgeons may have an ethical basis to decline nonemergent care if a potential patient indicates unwillingness to comply with essential postoperative treatments. Once doctors and surgeons, in particular, are in a relationship with a patient, there are obligations or responsibilities to treat that patient competently, respectfully, and tolerantly and not to neglect them. Physicians and surgeons, however, seem to be free to disengage from care for many reasons as long as they provide for actual or possible continuity of care if that is needed and desired by the patient.

Personal obligations to patients are just that. They can exist or be believed for many reasons. Membership in an extended family or a community may confer such an obligation. Training, specialty traditions, or even a particular role model or mentor may foster a special sense of obligation to all or a particular group of patients. A clinician's place in their medical career may alter their sense of obligation to patients and ability and opportunity to meet those obligations.

Personal obligations may stem from a deeply held spiritual or religious conviction. A passage from the Gospel of Saint Luke is a frequently cited example of such a conviction: "From everyone to whom much has been given, much will be required" (Luke 12:48). It is probably worth recalling for those who know it, and noting for those who do not, that Luke was a physician. Sacred texts are replete not only with obligations but with examples of noncompliance, albeit outside the medical domain. They provide a full spectrum of responses to noncompliance. The responses range from lethal punishment to forgiveness and reeducation. Noncompliance with religious practice or law is not the same as medical noncompliance, so one should be cautious before formulating a response based on nonanalagous situations.

What is meant and known about medical noncompliance?

Noncompliance, when it is used to describe behavior, generally denotes failure to follow an order, policy, or law. The implication is that the party whose behavior is in question has a legal, contractual, or contextual obligation to conform. Medical patients do not necessarily have this obligation. They have the prerogative to accept or reject medical recommendations for medical treatment, surgery, or changes in habits or behaviors. If they reject these recommendations, however, there may be serious consequences to their health and financial consequences to themselves and to others. Those others may also feel disrespect, disappointment, anger, frustration, and a sense of wasted effort or futility. The emotional reactions are intensified if patients fail to follow or adhere to recommendations or instructions to which they explicitly or tacitly agreed. It may be more accurate and helpful to physicians to identify this behavior as nonadherent because it clarifies that it is a departure from the patient's previous intent rather than a breach of a duty or an obligation to the physician.

Nonadherence is a prevalent human behavior. Just think of unfulfilled New Year's resolutions or health club memberships that go unused. The earliest physicians probably recognized medical nonadherence. Hippocrates wrote, "Keep watch also on the fault of patients which often make them lie about the taking of things prescribed" [15]. Nonadherence with medical regimens is quite common and has been documented to be about 50% with antihypertensive and even antituberculous therapy [16,17]. It has probably grown more common with the advent of drugs that are expensive, require multiple daily doses, and have unpleasant or dangerous side effects. Solid organ transplantation is an excellent example of the challenges that contemporary medical technology and surgery poses for patient adherence. Studies show that nonadherence with immunosuppressive therapy is common: 2% to 68% [18] for all organs and an average of 22% for kidney transplants [19]. Not surprisingly, it is associated with decreased graft survival and increased morbidity.

Although nonadherence is frequent, physicians generally presume adherence and fail to identify most nonadherent patients [20–22]. When they do identify such patients they often think of them as deviant or careless. It may be useful to acknowledge that clinicians too are often nonadherent and even noncompliant. In a hospital-based observational study of physicians' routine hand hygiene practices, Pittet and coworkers [23] found adherence averaged 57% and varied markedly across medical specialties. In multivariate analysis, adherence was associated with the awareness of being observed, the belief of being a role model for other colleagues, a positive attitude toward hand hygiene after patient contact, and easy access to hand-rub solution. Conversely, high workload, activities associated with a high risk for cross-transmission, and certain technical medical specialties (surgery, anesthesiology, emergency medicine, and intensive care medicine) were risk factors for nonadherence.

As that study of physician behavior shows, adherence or nonadherence is complex and multifactorial. Among patients, causes for nonadherence include misunderstanding; inability to comply (financial, physical, or physiologic); and not understanding the reason for a prescription or an action [15,24].

Predicting who is or will be nonadherent is perhaps even more complex and mostly counterintuitive. Poverty and poor education are not predictors. Age, gender, type of disease, and physician sociodemographic characteristics are weak and inconsistent predictors [15,21]. There are psychologic factors that do influence adherence but they are not fixed or easily identified before an illness or injury. They are situational and responsive. They include patients' levels of anxiety; motivation to recover; attitudes toward illness, treatment, and doctor; and the attitudes and beliefs of others including doctors in their environment [15].

When and why is nonadherence relevant?

Surgeons can respond differently to nonadherence if they identify it as an issue before they establish a relationship or operate, than if it occurs in the postoperative period. For example, if a patient refuses blood transfusion for an elective operation the surgeon can agree, perhaps alter the plan, explain the incumbent risks, acknowledge possible benefits, or arrange or suggest a referral to another more experienced or more willing surgeon. If a patient has a behavior or an addiction that could compromise the benefits of surgery, such as organ transplant, the surgeon and team could recommend changes, provide assistance in making them, and require a period of demonstrated adherence before proceeding with surgery. A recent history of nonadherence or addiction before a complex surgical procedure is worrisome, but not sufficient to preclude a patient from consideration. Many patients without that history prove to be nonadherent. Patients with that history who become adherent before surgery demonstrate some of the attitudinal and motivational factors that are associated with sustained adherence. Careful psychologic testing of all prospective transplant patients, not presumptive or stereotypical judgments, although not yet regarded as predictive may prove useful as a factor in counseling or selection [25,26]. Because donor organs are such a scarce resource, it seems justified to make anticipated adherence a criterion for eligibility. Because the consequences of ineligibility are so grave, however, judgment about adherence must be as careful, objective, and accurate as possible.

When nonadherence occurs after an operation, the surgeon faces different problems and has different strategies to use. Because not all nonadherence necessitates another operation, the medical response could come from clinicians responsible for some other aspect of the patient's care, such as cardiologists, infectious disease specialists, or transplant nurse-coordinators. If another operation is necessary but nonurgent and the patient desires it, the surgeon can use the strategies for preoperative nonadherence plus explore the reasons and circumstances that led to this result. Just as not all bad surgical outcomes result from surgeons' nonadherence to standards, not all bad outcomes result from patient nonadherence, even when it occurs. An operative site infection, intravenous catheter infection, or even donor organ failure may occur in a nonadherent patient but not because of the nonadherence. It is important to make the distinction, because patients who feel blamed for what they do not feel responsible for are likely to lose respect and trust in their physician, a critical factor for future adherence. If nonadherence clearly led to the need for surgery it is important to make that connection for the patient. It is equally important to investigate the reasons for it. If the patient was unable to purchase the requisite drugs, it does seem pointless to pursue a second procedure without resolving that problem, which may require the help of other professionals. If the patient has relapsed with an addiction, additional assistance and a period of abstinence are appropriate prerequisites to more surgery.

A particularly vexing problem for thoracic surgeons and for infectious disease physicians is a patient who uses illicit intravenous drugs and who has bacterial endocarditis. Although disturbing, this unlawful behavior, which really is noncompliant, does not excuse a surgeon from an obligation to perform a medically necessary operation. As has been seen, the obligation may not be generic, but it may arise from emergent circumstances, an established relationship, or a contractual commitment. An unobligated surgeon may still choose to proceed with surgery because he or she realizes that noncompliance with the law does not alter the grave prognosis of the infection or necessarily predict nonadherence or a poor surgical result. Studies on patients who are advised to seek help and overcome addictions show that, whereas some predictably fail or relapse, many succeed, in large part because of the factors mentioned previously and the assistance and encouragement of the medical team [25,27,28]. Surgeons often operate on presumed adherent patients with a disease, such as lung cancer, with a lower predicted 5-year survival than a valve replacement in an illicit drug user. The prognosis for the drug user is also more likely to reflect the skill and attitude of the team. Surgeons who decline to operate on such patients should be clear about their reasons and not confuse dislike or distaste for a patient or his or her behavior with a medical contraindication for surgery or with evidence that the surgery will certainly fail. They should also be clear about whether their medical concerns are short-term (ie, perioperative) or long-term, such as recurrent disease or other addiction-related problems. Evidence from patients with addictions to tobacco, alcohol, and illegal drugs may be helpful in this regard [25,27,29].

Does the surgeon have a special obligation to the nonadherent patient?

Because nonadherence is so common, so consequential, and so influenced by physicians, responsible surgeons have an incentive if not a duty to predict, prevent, identify, and manage it. Doing those things well reduces frustrations and produces better outcomes.

Prediction, although not precise, is better than prejudice or intuition. A history of nonadherence to a previous medical regimen, especially a similar one, is certainly a basis for concern. The concerned surgeon should share that concern directly and work with the patient and other professionals to establish and then reduce the risk of nonadherence or, if appropriate, postpone or cancel an operation.

Prevention by selection is a poor tool because there are few, if any, directly observable characteristics that allow a surgeon to screen out nonadherent patients. Prevention is also largely a function of the surgeon. Misunderstanding is preventable, but only if it is anticipated and identified early. Surgeons must communicate clearly and adapt to individual needs and abilities. Professional translators, support persons, written instructions, and pictures all help with understanding. The question, "do you understand," often does not help. If patients can explain to the clinician what they should do and why, then they understand. Otherwise one cannot know whether they understand. Prevention also depends on the surgeon's knowledge of the other essential elements of adherence: ability to pay, ability and means to get to treatment and appointments, and support persons who understand what is expected and are willing and able to help. If any of these elements are missing, steps to correct them may well prevent nonadherence.

Identifying nonadherence can be a challenge. There are false-negatives and false-positives. Clinicians overestimate adherence and often make unsupported assumptions about nonadherence. Unfortunately, if patients are asked about their adherence or are accused of nonadherence, they are being invited to lie. If it is acknowledged that adherence is hard for everyone and that at least some difficulty with complicated regimens is expected, an atmosphere in which it may be easier for some nonadherent patients to tell the truth is created. One should suspect, but not presume, nonadherence when the clinical course is not what is expected. Although other possibilities are pursued, it may be useful to have patients bring in their prescriptions to be sure they are correct, that they are labeled properly, to see how many pills have been taken, and when the prescription was filled. A physical examination for signs of tobacco or drug use and laboratory tests can be helpful when addiction is the concern.

Managing nonadherence may not be a technical skill acquired in training, or one that wins accolades from colleagues, but it can be the difference between a good surgeon or program as measured by outcomes and excellent ones. An article by the surgeon Gawande [30] makes that point about programs that treat cystic fibrosis. I suspect the same is true of heart transplant programs.

Summary

Professional oaths and codes do not establish a firm basis for the obligation to treat all patients and they provide little or no clear guidance about whether patient nonadherence exempts a physician from a specific contextual obligation to a patient. A long-standing and still prevalent tradition in surgery supports a strong obligation to one's established patients. A personal belief in an obligation to serve those less fortunate or even less compliant could support sustained treatment and special assistance to a nonadherent patient. A collective, professional, objective, informed decision to exclude a patient who is highly likely to be nonadherent or incapable of adherence from the benefit of a scarce resource, such as a human organ, is defensible and appropriate. A surgeon's decision to deny care to an established but nonadherent patient is much less so. Adherence is as dependent on physician attitude, skill, and behavior as it is on patients' nonadherence. To the degree that it reflects less than competent management of this prevalent problem, it can be considered an error or complication that makes most surgeons feel even more obliged to mitigate or rectify the problem. This article describes the almost ubiquitous phenomenon of nonadherence; a way to reconceptualize noncompliance; and practical steps that can help predict, prevent, identify, and manage it. It is hoped that this helps surgeons reduce the frequency of nonadherence, make dealing with it less onerous, and consequently achieve better outcomes.

It is reasonable to think about nonadherence in terms of three roles. The surgeon's role is to make the patient's choice informed, to be aware of the risk factors for nonadherence, and not make adherence any more difficult than it has to be. The patient's role is to make choices between value-laden alternatives. Society's role is equitably to distribute scarce medical resources to patients who can and want to adhere to the necessary regimen to benefit from them [31].

Acknowledgments

Linda Carr-Lee and Natalie Burbank provided valuable research and editorial assistance and manuscript preparation.

References

[1] Edelstein L. Translation from the Greek. In: Edelstein L, editor. The Hippocratic Oath: text, translation, and interpretation. Baltimore: Johns Hopkins Press; 1943.

[2] Gabriel BA. Oath of Lasagna (1964). In: A Hippocratic Oath for our time. American Association of Medical Colleges. September 2001. Available at: www.aamc.org/newsroom/reporter/sept2001/hippocraticoath.htm. Accessed May 28, 2005.

[3] The Oath of Maimonides. In: Halsall P, editor. Internet history sourcebooks project. Available at: http://www.fordham.edu/halsall/source/rambam-oath.html. Accessed May 28, 2005.

[4] Gabriel BA. Declaration of Geneva (World Medical Association 1948). In: A Hippocratic Oath for our time. American Association of Medical Colleges. September 2001. Available at: www.aamc.org/newsroom/reporter/sept2001/hippocraticoath.htm. Accessed May 28, 2005.

[5] Gabriel BA. A Hippocratic Oath for Our Time. American Association of Medical Colleges. September 2001. Available at: www.aamc.org/newsroom/reporter/sept2001/hippocraticoath.htm. Accessed May 28, 2005.

[6] American Medical Association. Code of Ethics, adopted May, 1847. Philadelphia: Turner-Hamilton; 1871.

[7] Council on Ethical and Judicial Affairs. Code of Medical Ethics: Current opinions with annotations. American Medical Association: 2002: 286. Available at: http://www.ama-assn.org/ama/pub/category/2498.html. Accessed May 28, 2005.

[8] Council on Ethical and Judicial Affairs. Code of Medical Ethics: Current opinions with annotations. American Medical Association: 2002: XIV. Available at: http://www.ama-assn.org/ama/pub/category/2512.html. Accessed May 28, 2005.

[9] Council on Ethical and Judicial Affairs. Code of Medical Ethics: Current opinions with annotations. American Medical Association: 2002: 289. Available at: http://www.ama-assn.org/ama/pub/category/2512.html. Accessed May 28, 2005.

[10] Council on Ethical and Judicial Affairs. Code of Medical Ethics: Current opinions with annotations. American Medical Association: 2002: 217. Available at: http://www.ama-assn.org/ama/pub/category/2512.html. Accessed May 28, 2005.

[11] American College of Surgeons, preamble. Avaliable at: http://www.facs.org/fellows_info/statements/stonprin.html#pre. Accessed May 28, 2005.

[12] American College of Surgeons, Code of Professional Conduct. Available at: http://www.facs.org/fellows_info/statements/stonprin.html#pre. Accessed May 28, 2005.

[13] American College of Surgeons, Qualifications of the Responsible Surgeon, Competencies. Available at: http://www.facs.org/fellows_info/statements/stonprin.html#pre. Accessed May 28, 2005.

[14] American College of Surgeons, Relation of the Surgeon to the Patient. Available at: http://www.facs.org/fellows_info/statements/stonprin.html#pre. Accessed May 28, 2005.

[15] Evans L, Spelman M. The problem of non-compliance with drug therapy. Drugs 1983;25:63–76.

[16] Costa FV. Compliance with anti-hypertensive treatment. Clin Exp Hypertens 1996;18:463–72.

[17] Dixon WM, Stradling P, Woolton DP. Outpatient PAS therapy. Lancet 1957;2:871–2.

[18] Butler JA, Roderick P, Mullee M, et al. Frequency and impact of nonadherence to immunosuppressants after renal transplantation: a systematic review. Transplantation 2004;77:769–76.

[19] Chisholm MA. Issues of adherence to immunosuppressant therapy after solid-organ transplantation. Drugs 2002;62:567–75.
[20] Wright EC. Non-compliance—or how many ants has Matilda? Lancet 1993;342:909–13.
[21] Stephenson BJ, Rowe BH, Haynes RB, et al. Is this patient taking the treatment as prescribed? JAMA 1993;269:2779–81.
[22] Melinkow J, Kiefe C. Patient compliance and medical research: issues in methodology. J Gen Intern Med 1994;9:96–105.
[23] Pittet D, Simon A, Hugonnet S, et al. Hand hygiene among physicians: performance, beliefs, and perceptions. Ann Intern Med 2004;141:1–8.
[24] Fletcher RH. Patient compliance with therapeutic advice: a modern view. Mt Sinai J Med 1989;56:453–8.
[25] Maxson PM, Schultz KL, Berge KH, et al. Probable alcohol abuse or dependence: a risk factor for intensive-care readmission in patients undergoing elective vascular and thoracic surgical procedures. May Perioperative Outcomes Group. Mayo Clin Proc 1999;74:448–53.
[26] Shapiro PA, Williams DL, Foray AT, et al. Psychosocial evaluation and prediction of compliance problems and morbidity after heart transplantation. Transplantation 1995;60:1462–6.
[27] Dresler CM, Bailey M, Roper CR, et al. Smoking cessation and lung cancer resection. Chest 1996;110:1199–202.
[28] Bellamy CO, DiMartini AM, Ruppert K, et al. Liver transplantation for alcoholic cirrhosis: long term follow-up and impact of disease recurrence. Transplantation 2001;72:619–26.
[29] Hanrahan JS, Eberly C, Mohanty PK. Substance abuse in heart transplant recipients: a 10-year follow-up study. Prog Transplant 2001;11:285–90.
[30] Gawande A. The bell curve: what happens when patients find out how good their doctors really are. The New Yorker December 6, 2004;80:82–95.
[31] Jacobson JA. Compliance and adherence. In: Sugarman J, editor. Twenty common problems: ethics in primary care. New York: McGraw-Hill; 2000. p. 39–48.

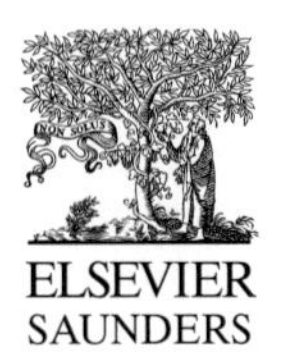
ELSEVIER
SAUNDERS

Thorac Surg Clin 15 (2005) 469 – 480

THORACIC
SURGERY
CLINICS

Withdrawing Life-Sustaining Treatment: Ethical Considerations

Sharon Reynolds, RN, BA, BScN, MHSc[a,b,*], Andrew B. Cooper, MD, MHSc[c,d], Martin McKneally, MD, PhD[a]

[a]*Joint Centre for Bioethics, University of Toronto, 88 College Street, Toronto, Ontario M5G 1L4, Canada*
[b]*Medical-Surgical Intensive Care Unit, Toronto General Hospital, 585 University Avenue, Toronto, Ontario M5G 2N2, Canada*
[c]*The Interdisciplinary Division of Critical Care Medicine, University of Toronto, Toronto, Ontario, Canada*
[d]*Sunnybrook and Women's College Health Sciences Centre, M3-200, 2075 Bayview Avenue, Toronto, Ontario M4N 3M5, Canada*

Withdrawing life-supporting technology from patients who are irremediably ill is morally troubling for caregivers, patients, and families. Interventions that enable clinicians to delay death create situations in which the dignity and comfort of dying patients may be sacrificed to spare professionals and families from their elemental fear of death. Understanding of the limits of treatment, expertise in palliation of symptoms, skillful communication, and careful orchestration of controllable events can help to manage the withdrawal of life support appropriately.

Case illustration

You have known your patient Sid for a long time; it seems forever. For 6 months, following an esophagectomy for cancer, his course has been marked by severe complications. Necrosis at the gastroesophageal anastomosis led to an enterocutaneous fistula. Ten subsequent operations and multiple consultants have failed to improve his condition. His chest wall drains continuously, and he has lost 42 pounds. During physiotherapy he despondently told his nurse "I just want to die." Not long after, he developed pneumonia and was transferred back to the ICU for mechanical ventilation. Two days later, you agreed with his wife and son that a do-not-resuscitate order is appropriate. After a trial of therapy on the ventilator for 2 weeks, the family asked you to call a halt to the life support including vasoactive therapy, antibiotics, and mechanical ventilation. Although Sid was not a capable decision-maker at this point, their feeling was that his earlier statements of despair justified their decision on his behalf.

Why is withdrawal of life support so hard to do?

Because technology has become so effective at extending life, it is difficult to determine when it is appropriate to accept that a patient is dying, cease further aggressive treatment, and strengthen palliative support. A host of issues contribute to the difficulty of withdrawing life-sustaining treatments: the distinction between withholding and withdrawing treatment, religious and cultural considerations, the technologic imperative, prognostic uncertainty, variability in practice, and caregiver discomfort with death. This article focuses on the withdrawal of life-sustaining treatment, because this is the more problematic area for health care providers.

* Corresponding author. Joint Centre for Bioethics, University of Toronto, 88 College Street, Toronto, Ontario M5G IL4, Canada.
E-mail address: sharon.reynolds@utoronto.ca (S. Reynolds).

1547-4127/05/$ – see front matter
doi:10.1016/j.thorsurg.2005.06.002

Withdrawing versus withholding life support

Despite consensus that there is no ethical or legal distinction between withholding and withdrawing treatment [1–6], caregivers experience a disturbing difference between the two in practice [5,7–9]. The determining factor is the need for human agency in withdrawal. A trusted and responsible member of the care team must take action and disconnect the ventilator or turn off the inotropic medications supporting blood pressure. This action may lead to immediate death. The feeling of responsibility and culpability for the death that follows is almost inescapable despite theoretical distinctions, professional endorsements, and legal precedents. Seymour [8] followed ICU physicians on their daily rounds and observed their end-of-life decision-making processes. Unless the patient was very close to death, physicians were not comfortable withdrawing support even though they had earlier acknowledged a grim prognosis. They believed they were justified in withdrawing treatment only when "it becomes clear that death will occur in spite of any further treatment maneuvers. In this way a causative link between non-treatment and death is avoided."

To withdraw life support is to recognize that the underlying disease process cannot be reversed. The intention is not to kill, although death certainly ensues. The intention is to acknowledge the limits of medicine. The death that follows, even if immediate, indicates the severity of the disease state and uncovers the inability of the patient's body to survive. Life-support measures mask this reality, but the routine interventions that cannot reverse the underlying disease process may confuse families, who often associate ongoing treatment with hope for recovery. Care-related activities that focus on intravenous drips, monitoring lines, and equipment are consoling routines for caregivers even as death becomes inevitable and disease "overmasters the patient." Withdrawal in this setting is a courageous but distressing act of kindness.

Religious and cultural considerations

Religious views may influence decisions to withdraw life-sustaining treatments. It is important to determine the religious beliefs held by the patient or family. One needs to know what their beliefs mean in the context of the present situation. If they are uncertain, yet they wish to adhere to the tenets of their chosen religion, they may need to consult a religious representative within that tradition. Belonging to a specific faith community does not necessarily mean that the patient subscribes to all or any of the tenets of that faith. Most religious outlooks on life share a belief in the sanctity of human life, as a gift from God. Sanctity of life may mean different things to different people. Life has supreme value, for example, in Orthodox Jewish tradition. In this view, withdrawal of supportive therapies is not permissible unless the patient's death, defined by cessation of the heartbeat, is imminent [10–12]. Life-sustaining treatments that are available should be sought [13,14]. Quality-of-life arguments supporting withdrawal of care have no meaning in this context, because the quality of one's life does not define the value of a human being. Within this perspective tube feeding a patient in a persistent vegetative state is morally obligatory care unless the patient is deemed terminally ill (terminal illness in Jewish law is understood as a life expectancy of 3 months [14]) and considered to be suffering. Brain death, as a definition of the termination of life, is not universally accepted [15]. It is very difficult for some people to be told that their loved one is dead yet he or she has a pulse and a blood pressure [16,17].

Religious views are thought to underlie the observation that physicians from Greece, Italy, and Portugal are less inclined to withdraw life-sustaining treatments. "Physicians with a Catholic background were less likely to withhold and withdraw therapy than their Protestant or agnostic counterparts" [18].

Attitudes among laypersons toward life-sustaining interventions were surveyed with scenario questionnaires. Korean Americans believe that life support should always be considered even though this is not what they would choose for themselves. African Americans believe that life-sustaining interventions could be forgone, yet they themselves want such interventions. Within the Chinese culture it is considered rude and courting bad luck to disclose a fatal diagnosis to a patient, obviating direct discussion of withdrawal [19]. Health care providers can initiate conversation that reveals these personal belief systems to guide clinicians in how to speak to patients and what treatments to provide.

Technology: a moral obligation

Significant advances in medical technology and the treatment of disease have changed the goal of medicine from treating what can be treated and respecting what cannot be treated to one of combating death [20]. Technology can be seductive. It can create the illusion of providing certainty and reducing ambiguity. "Like the broom in The Sorcerer's Apprentice, technologies come to have a life of their own..." [21], transforming and dehumanizing the dying process.

The technical components of clinical practice and the myriad interventions possible in a given patient's care represent what can be done to hold death at bay. The question of what ought to be done is grounded in value systems. Disagreements about the right thing to do that arise in this meeting place between value systems and technology can often be reconciled through ethics consultation.

The availability of technology may create a sense of moral obligation to use it based on a belief that to treat is to care. In contrast, clinicians feel responsible, even culpable, if they choose to use technology and then withdraw it. This reasoning leads one to value technology more "than competent compassionate care at the end of life..." [22]. In some ways the intuitive and clinically rooted notions of what is happening to the body of a patient are not trusted. Clinicians feel morally obligated to continue technologic support despite unlikely survival. "Whereas nature once decided who would live or die, our technological capacities have come to play that role" [20] in resource-rich countries. Where there are fewer technologic resources, end-of-life decisions are made with less certainty and conflict.

Prognostic uncertainty

Uncertainty contributes to the dominance of technology in medicine [21]. Decisions to withdraw therapy are based on predictions of future events, deduced from general rules applied to an individual who may not fit that generalization precisely. Because a decision to withdraw treatment becomes irreversible when death occurs, prognostic uncertainty is less tolerable than it is in other domains of medical practice. Prognostic tools, such as Apache II to predict survival probability, do not "provide sufficient power to discriminate accurately between non-survivors and survivors" [23]. When Apache II scores were used with ICU patients on day 1 of admission, "the false positive prediction rate was 7.6% (9 of 118)." A positive prediction rate of 92.4%, although high, does not eliminate the risk of error. In another investigation of predictors of death in critical care units, treatment was withdrawn from 166 patients who were predicted by physicians to die. Six (3.6%) patients in this group eventually left hospital [24]. When compared with validated outcome prediction rules, the physician's own prediction of an adverse prognostic or cognitive function outcome, rather than a score, was the strongest predictor of death. The irreducible nature of uncertainty should not prevent accomplishing a right action. Instead it brings a duty to reflect with the family on the low probability of survival and the poor quality and short duration of residual life.

Physicians generally deal with uncertainty by choosing a course that maximizes potential benefit and minimizes the risk of complications or death. "Clinicians help families by acknowledging prognostic uncertainty directly and by building on that uncertainty to expand the discussion beyond an exclusive focus on survival" [25].

Variability in practice

In addition to uncertainty about outcomes, variabilities in the practice of withdrawing life support are "caused by the idiosyncratic values, beliefs and habits of individual physicians" [8]. Even when physicians use the best evidence available, "their own ethical, social, moral, and religious values influence their medical decision making" [26]. Most Pennsylvania physicians chose to withdraw therapy so that death occurs in subsequent days rather than immediately. Diagnostic uncertainty was a potent factor in the decision. When uncertainty was not a concern, most physicians chose death in 15 minutes over death in 4 hours. Other important factors influencing decision making in this study were defensive motivation (physicians were less likely to withdraw a treatment supporting an organ system that had failed because of iatrogenic complications) and duration of prior therapy. Physicians were less likely to withdraw therapies that had been in place for a long time [27]. Underlining the idiosyncratic and seemingly arbitrary decision-making process regarding withdrawal, a survey of Canadian critical care physicians found that, "in only one of 12 scenarios did more than 50% of the respondents make the same treatment choice" [26].

Legal perspectives

Legal recourse is a last resort when differences of opinion about withdrawing life-sustaining treatment cannot be resolved by other means. The courts tend to support the autonomous rights of patients or their surrogates to make decisions consistent with the value systems of the patients.

In the case of Nancy B., the court faced a conflict when asked to honor the autonomous decision-making rights of a competent patient asking to be disconnected from a ventilator that was sustaining her life. The right to refuse life-sustaining treatment is embodied in the legal doctrine of informed consent [4]. Nancy B. was a 25-year-old woman who had suffered from Guillain-Barré disease for 2.5 years. The conflict in this case existed between a patient's autonomous right to refuse life-sustaining treatments and Section 14 of the Criminal Code, which states that no person may consent to an act that results in their death. The Criminal Code equated withdrawal with euthanasia. This prohibits physicians from ever withdrawing treatment. Mr. Justice Dufour of the Quebec Superior Court needed to find a way to reconcile this conflict. He did so not by interpreting Nancy B.'s request as a request for physician-assisted suicide "but, rather, as an attempt merely to allow a disease to take its natural course" [28]. This case establishes in law that it is the underlying disease that causes the death, not the physician who withdraws unwanted life-supporting treatment.

The case of Helga Wanglie provided further evidence of court support for the decision-making rights of the patient with her husband acting as her surrogate. Helga Wanglie was an 87-year-old woman who had developed pneumonia and respiratory failure following hip replacement surgery. Five months later she suffered a cardiac arrest and never regained consciousness. In June 1990, 1 month after her arrest, physicians sought court permission to discontinue her ventilatory support because Helga could not be weaned from the ventilator and was believed to be in a persistent vegetative state. Her husband argued that physicians are not God and "Only He who gave life has the right to take life." The court supported Mr. Wanglie as best able to represent his wife's interests. Helga died 7 days after the court decision [29]. Current practice supports respecting value systems and beliefs that honor sanctity of life. As resource constraints increase, these issues will be debated publicly.

Physicians made a unilateral decision to place a do-not-resuscitate order on the chart of 72-year-old Catherine Gilgunn, against the wishes of her daughter. The patient's medical history included diabetes, heart disease, Parkinson's disease, and cerebrovascular disease. Refractory seizures had rendered her irreversibly comatose. Hospital lawyers supported the decision of the physician to instate a do-not-resuscitate order despite disagreement from the patient's daughter. The decision was believed to be in the "patient's best interests." When her daughter took legal action against her mother's physicians and the hospital, the Superior Court of Massachusetts supported the medical team. The physicians argued that their decision to withhold nonbeneficial treatment was "consistent with professional standards" [30]. Despite this finding by the court, unilateral decision making is not recommended [31,32], especially in withdrawal of life support.

Recently, Laura Hawryluck, an intensive care physician, asked permission of the court to remove the daughters of her patient as decision makers for their irreversibly demented mother who has required repeated admissions to the ICU for ventilatory support during recurrent bouts of pneumonia. Given the frequent dependence on ICU intervention and the inability to reverse the underlying disease process, Dr. Hawryluck asked for permission to focus on palliative support on a hospital ward instead of ICU care. The court ruled against Dr. Hawryluck, supporting the request of the family for ICU care consistent with their mother's religious views (a link to the Hawryluck case is http://www.canlii.org/on/cas/onsc/2004/2004onsc10339.html).

Can physicians refuse to provide care that is clearly prolonging death and not of benefit? Perhaps "terminally ill patients do not have the right to demand any and all treatments" [33]. There are guidelines provided by the American Thoracic Society and the Society of Critical Care Medicine regarding the withdrawal of treatment in situations considered futile. A physician is not morally obligated to initiate or continue a treatment considered not to be of benefit to a patient or to yield a quality of life not acceptable to the patient. It is suggested that consent of the patient or surrogate decision maker is not required [34–36]. Proceeding without consent remains legally problematic.

Downie [32] argues that there is "an urgent need for lawmakers to clarify when doctors have the right to withhold and withdraw their services." Health care providers are currently stuck in a gray zone on these issues.

The withdrawal process: how to do it

Because withdrawal of life support typically happens when patients have become incapable of communicating directly with clinicians, the process usually involves substitute decision making with the patient's family [25]. Estimates of the proportion of patients involved in decision making under these circumstances vary in the literature from 6% to 35% [37,38]. Few critically ill patients arrive in the ICU with explicit advance directives [39] and, where present, the language of an advanced care directive may lack power to address the particulars of the patient's circumstances. Even if an advance directive exists, the personal values it reflects may change in altered circumstances. Preferences in the new situation cannot be assumed to be identical to those in an advance directive. Despite a reasonable likelihood of success for resuscitative therapy, patients modify their choices in light of the accompanying disability. As the burden of disability increases, fewer patients choose to be resuscitated [40]. Empirical data underlie the importance of meticulous informed consent for high-risk surgical procedures. Beyond the usual discussion of postoperative complications, the possibility of a prolonged ICU stay with its attendant burdens of suffering [41] should be discussed, including an exploration of the patient's preferences should survival with severe disability be the outcome. A well-documented preoperative discussion of patient preferences when considering withdrawal of life support in the context of anticipated degrees of disability can inform action in the patient's best interest. One of us (MM) has engaged in this practice for many years. Most patients are grateful for the opportunity to discuss this possibility. A small number are unable to address it, because they are already overwhelmed by thinking about their illness and its treatment.

Although there are rare circumstances in which it may be possible to awaken critically ill patients to discuss treatment options, this is usually not practical. Sepsis itself may impair capacity and severe hypoxemia that accompanies respiratory failure in critical illness makes reversal of sedative medication effects problematic, mainly because of the difficulty in maintaining patient ventilator synchrony. Hepatic and renal dysfunction, altered volumes of distribution, and reduced protein binding may delay clearance of centrally acting drugs. The obligation to involve patients in their care decisions, based on the principle of respect for persons, must be balanced against the suffering that removal of sedation and analgesia may cause during a terminal critical illness [42].

Communication with families of critically ill patients about withdrawal of life support is not easy. A useful reflective taxonomy is to consider physician, environmental, and family factors contributing to inadequate communication. There is a growing literature on the inadequacy of physician communication in this setting. When family conferences are studied, physicians dominate the discussion. In some instances, up to 70% of the content is uttered by the physician. There are frequent physician-induced turns of conversation [43]. Physicians miss opportunities in about one third of family conferences to be empathic, to listen to family concerns, and to address key principles of palliative care [44].

Ideally, responsible staff physicians should conduct family conferences in the presence of house staff and nurses. Families of patients find information conveyed by junior staff less satisfactory and less understandable compared with discussions held with attending physicians. They are likely to require additional communication if the initial contact is by a junior doctor [45]. Compared with satisfaction with nurse communication, family satisfaction with physician communication is modest but improves as the number of physician visits increases [46]. "The virtue of being present" is a theme expressed throughout the literature on withdrawal of life support in the ICU and elsewhere in palliative care medicine. Families of critically ill patients are often overwhelmed by exposure to the information-dense environment of the ICU and their concern for a loved one. The prevalence of anxiety and depression is high, reaching nearly 70% when both symptoms are considered together [47]. Emotional distress may interfere with capacity of family members to act as substitute decision makers. Families are more likely to experience effective communication when it is conducted in a private conference room than when sensitive discussions are conducted in public places like hallways. The bedside in the ICU is unsuitable; there is a high likelihood of interruptions and distractions [48] and paroxysmal noise levels sometimes exceeding 70 dB [49], the equivalent of busy street corners.

Communication with distressed families to discuss limits of treatment requires specialized skills and attitudes on the part of the physician. Although many of these skills are in the domain of social workers, hospital chaplains, or bioethicists, the attending surgeon or physician is medically and legally responsible and accountable for decisions about treatment.

Essential skills include the ability to establish trust, to appreciate affective moments and show empathy, and to communicate medical facts in nontechnical language. Ideally, the surgeon engages family decision makers in a dialog about reasonable treatment options, reflective of the goals and health-related values of the patient; the deliberative physician patient relationship is most appropriate when there is adequate time and commitment [50]. The importance of relationship as a vehicle for creating trust means that arriving at a shared plan takes time and commitment to ongoing dialog. The empathic response to expressions of emotion is to state simply that one has noticed the emotion and to express acceptance and appreciation that it is appropriate [51].

During family conferences, silence is often more valuable than words. When disagreements emerge among family members or between the health care team and the family in a conference, deliberately allowing silence to develop is an excellent way to refocus the discussion. Silence in the context of empathic communication gives the patient's family the experience of being understood [52]. Silence enlightens and enlivens ethical reflection.

Dealing with requests for euthanasia

Four hours after extubation, the bedside nurse calls you to express her concern that Sid is struggling for air. She tells you that in 11 years of ICU nursing she has never witnessed so much suffering in a dying patient. "He seems to be indestructible. I cannot imagine what it will take to end his suffering, unless it's something like KCL." The family at the bedside looks up at you despairingly.

Outside critical care settings, surveys in the United States, Britain, and Australia reveal that about one quarter of physicians and nurses are approached by patients or families at some time with requests for active euthanasia or physician-assisted death. Of these respondents, a small proportion accommodates the requests. Within critical care units, one survey of a random sample of 1600 nurses subscribing to the journal *Nursing* (readership 500,000) revealed that 17% had received such requests. Of those who received requests, 16% accommodated them, sometimes by pretending to provide life-sustaining treatment while omitting it. The investigators estimated that about 7% of nurses involved in these activities initiated them without the knowledge of decision makers, claiming tacit consent [53]. Without clear guidance on quality end-of-life care, idiosyncratic solutions are the norm.

A combination of factors, such as nonacceptance of death, the virtuous desire to relieve suffering, and lack of confidence in the training and ability of physicians to control symptoms at the end of life, lead to the conclusion that the only solution seems to be active euthanasia. A study of 36 patients followed by a university palliative care service revealed only about two thirds of patients rated their care as very good or excellent [54]. The same investigators found that priorities for improvement were in domains of symptom control (pain, shortness of breath, thirst, and other symptoms); reducing delays (in care, diagnosis, and transfer home); better access to their physicians and nurses (for information and improved therapeutic alliances); and the addressing of emotional concerns, such as loneliness and fear of abandonment. Quantification of the quality of death is possible and offers insight into what can be done to improve the practice of withdrawal of life support. A systematically developed measurement tool quality of death and dying highlights key patient-identified preferences for end-of-life care [55]. The quality of death in the ICU falls far short of what is valued by dying patients. Palliative care in the ICU differs from care in other settings, because the dying process is more dramatic or linked to medical decision-making, and because the time from initiation of the process to death is usually shorter. There are special problems in the assessment of pain and suffering in ICU patients: communication problems, severity of illness, decreased levels of consciousness, and difficulty interpreting the usual clinical signs of distress [56].

The focus in the practice of withdrawal of life support should be on those items that can be changed; symptom control (pain and dyspnea); preparation for death (supporting the family and offering spiritual care); the conduct of death (inviting family to be present); ending unwanted therapies; and encouraging physical contact as the transition occurs. Palliative care initiatives can address the shortcomings that bring about requests for active euthanasia and physician assisted death in critically ill patients.

Symptom control during withdrawal of life support

You return to the bedside, where Sid is gasping for breath. His systolic blood pressure is 50 mm Hg, and despite high doses of midazolam (320 mg) and an increase in the hydromorphone infusion to 500 mg/h he still is apparently in severe distress.

Physicians attempting to relieve symptoms in dying patients tread a difficult path; if not enough medication is given, there is the risk of inadequate symptom control. If too much is given, there is the risk of being accused of practicing active euthanasia or physician-assisted death. The dosages mentioned previously were administered to a dying patient in Canada. Responding to the distress of the patient, his family, and the bedside nurse, a physician decided to hasten death with medication devoid of analgesic or anxiolytic effect: potassium chloride. In the testimony of expert witnesses during an inquiry to determine whether the physician would be committed to stand trial for first-degree murder, drug dosages were a focus of testimony. Two days before the patient's death, procedural pain during an incision and drainage had been relieved with only fractions of the previously mentioned amounts: 5 mg of hydromorphone and 2 mg of midazolam. The patient's body was exhumed in the investigation, but a toxicology report found only "traces of dilaudid and morphine in the liver." A critical care physician who testified pointed out that the apparent ineffectiveness of such large doses of medication should have prompted an investigation of the effectiveness of the intravenous access used to administer medications for symptom control [57]. The first practice point in symptom control during withdraw of life support is to review the medication history, determining the treatments in use and the patient's responses both at rest and during stimulation. This guides the practitioner toward an appropriate starting point for symptom control. Next, inspection of the intravenous access is important. In edematous patients it may be difficult to determine whether existing peripheral intravenous lines are intravascular or interstitially placed. If there is doubt, it is prudent to replace them or to ensure they are functioning appropriately before relying on them in withdrawing life support. Injecting a bolus of a marker, such as a rapidly cleared vasoactive drug (eg, phenylephrine, 100 μg, if not contraindicated), may help to clarify the adequacy of existing catheters without the delay associated with acquiring a drug level. If this step is necessary, perhaps because of excessive difficulty or risk associated with replacement of existing intravenous access, it is important explicitly to declare the intention associated with the injection of the marker dose in the orders and the patient care record. When writing orders for symptom control it is important to specify indications for all comfort medications to avoid the potential for accusations of assisted euthanasia or physician-assisted death (eg, by writing "for pain and dyspnea" after the opioid and "for anxiety" after the benzodiazepine dosages).

Guidelines on the use of medication in these settings are helpful to maintain practice within the standards of the profession. Table 1 summarizes key points of the statement on end-of-life care of the Society of Critical Care Medicine, and of a Delphi study systematically evaluating the consensus of Canadian Intensive Care specialists, and provincial coroners [56]. The Society of Critical Care Medicine recommendations present a useful taxonomy for commonly encountered scenarios in withdrawal of ventilatory support [58]. It classifies the needs of patients according to neurologic function and the like-

Table 1
Management of pain and suffering

Relief of pain and suffering	Nonpharmacologic means Ensure presence of friends, family, pastoral care Change technologic environment	Pharmacologic means Analgesics, sedatives, adjuncts Treat pain, suffering or both with appropriate agents
Initial dosages	Invidualize Therapy ∝ Narcotic exposure, age, prior alcohol, drug use Organ dysfunction Level of consciousness Level of psychologic support Wishes for sedation during death	See below for summary of pharmacology
Titration of sedatives and analgesics	Increase doses in response to signs Doses may exceed preconceived notions Patient's request Tachycardia, hypertension, sweating Facial grimacing, tears, vocalization with movement Restlessness	Limitations of clinical indicators Imprecise Supplement with VAS pain, RASS scale
Maximum doses	Maximum doses do not exist[a] If specified, some patients may suffer with inadequate symptom control	The intent of the treating physician distinguishes palliative care from AE, PAD
Pre-emptive or responsive therapy?	Clear documentation of intention is required	Pre-emptive dosing in anticipation of pain or suffering is good palliative care, not AE

Abbreviations: AE, active euthanasia; PAD, physician assisted death; RASS, Richmond agitation-sedation scale; VAS, visual analogue scale.

[a] In one case series of terminal weaning of chronic ventilator-dependent patients, morphine doses given during withdraw of life support ranged from 2–50 mg and benzodiazepine doses ranged from 8–675 mg.

Table 2
Anticipation and treatment of discomfort in withdrawal of life support

Neurologic function	Likelihood of distress	Technique
Brain death	None; possibility of lazarus reflexes	Extubation; preparation of family
Comatose patients	Uncertain	Extubation or rapid ↓ support; ± sedation
Conscious patients	High	Gradual ↓support; titrate sedation

lihood of dyspnea. There are three possibilities, and the approach to symptom control should be adapted accordingly (Table 2).

Symptom control in paralyzed patients

Many of the signs of pain and suffering in dying patients are masked by neuromuscular paralysis. Canadian and American expert opinion concurs that the use of neuromuscular blockade to mask the signs of death or to initiate withdraw of life support while neuromuscular blockade is still present is unethical [56,58,59]. Even under optimal conditions it is hard to monitor and correctly interpret bedside tests of neuromuscular function. Pre-emptive treatment of pain and suffering is appropriate if patients have been receiving neuromuscular blockade and continue to manifest paralysis despite discontinuation of drug infusions.

Conflict resolution and family demands for inappropriate treatment

It is normal for conflicts to occur at the end of life. Accepting this allows the team to look at conflict from a broader perspective. Death of the person becomes a prominent part of illness narratives before death of the physical body [60]. The stages of the grieving process, which in premodern times occurred after death, are displaced by life support to the period before death. Grief can be expressed through conflict in discussions about the futility of treatment as the family encounters and struggles with the impending loss of their beloved.

Families have the opportunity to discuss care with a diversity of teams in the ICU. The composition and structure of these teams is complex and their membership frequently changes. Differences in sensitivity

Box 1. Accepting conflict and creating dialogue

Ask the family:

- What do you understand about what is going on?
- Why have you decided to _____?
- What are you hoping we can accomplish/achieve?
- What do you think _____ would want us to accomplish for him/her?
- What else would he/she want us to accomplish?
- Which, of these, are the most important?
- In what situations, if any, could you imagine _____ not wanting to continue to live?
- Are your questions getting answered? Do you have concerns about the care you/your loved one is getting?
- Are there disagreements among family members?

Ask yourself:

- What do I think are this patient's chances of surviving to discharge recovering function?
- What have I told the patient/family are his/her chances of surviving to discharge/recovering function?
- How sure am I about his/her prognosis? On what is it based?
- What do I know about what this patient wants or would have wanted? How do I know? How sure am I?
- Is this patient competent to make his/her own decisions? How do I know? How sure am I? Could it be fluctuating or reversible incompetence?
- Did I/we contribute to a bad outcome in any way (eg, missed diagnosis, delayed treatment)?
- How do I feel about discussing this patient's death with him/her (his/her family)?

Who is this patient's ''family doctor''? Clergy of choice? Primary nurse? Social worker?
Do I feel I have enough time to talk to the patient/family about prognosis, options, and goals?
What words or phrases have I (for others) used that might be contributing to the conflict (eg, ''stopping treatment,'' ''comfort measures only,'' ''hopeless,'' ''certain'')?
What aspectist of this patient's life do I feel justify withholding or withdrawing life-sustaining treatment?
Does the family trust us? If not, why not?

Ask about social/ organizational influences:
Are there financial pressures on the family?
Are there financial pressures on the hospital?
Are there financial pressures on the medical team?
Are families allowed to see what the patient's day is like?
Are there any concerns about malpractice or legality?
Are there cultural or religious differences among the patient/ family/physicians/hospital?

From Goold SD, Williams B, Arnold RM. Conflicts regarding decisions to limit treatment: a differential diagnosis. JAMA 2000;283:909–14; with permission.

to the needs of families may bring about conflict. Continuity and consistency in communication is often difficult to maintain. Physicians in the ICU do not communicate well with each other. They miss opportunities for direct communication and use intermediaries, such as trainees or the chart, for important messages. Leaving a consulting service "out of the loop" with regard to the content of important family conferences can result in the communication of inconsistent messages to families. Families struggle with difficult personal, emotional, or religious aspects, whereas teams encounter challenges in regard to their authority in the decision-making process. Shared medical responsibility among several teams leads to problems in giving clear guidance to families. Families, who may value intensive care as an expression of devotion to the person or as part of religious duty, are confused and offended when team members seem to undervalue their technologic interventions based on medical effectiveness.

A series of penetrating questions that explore family, physician, and institutional or social influences contributing to the conflict is discussed in a scheme for the differential diagnosis of conflicts as outlined in Box 1 [61]. This scheme for differential diagnosis presents a useful framework for the exploration of the family's experience of illness and opens the door to the creation of a therapeutic narrative in which their experience is acknowledged and validated. It also gives guidelines for the physician, highlighting areas in which support may be needed.

Summary

In the community of caregivers, there is a general consensus that some heroic measures are not obligatory in certain circumstances that are defined by professional norms. For example, cardiopulmonary resuscitation in terminal cancer patients is not endorsed because of its violation of the dignity of the irremediably ill, and its unproductive cost to society. Moving back from this extreme, the availability and effectiveness of life-prolonging treatments, such as ventilators, dialysis, and implantable mechanical hearts, moves into a domain where the boundary limit of the obligation to preserve life is less clearly defined. When the continuing intervention of caregivers is essential to the prolongation of life, but the outcome and quality of residual life has deteriorated far below everyone's expectations when the treatment was initiated, caregivers are morally troubled as their treatments prolong the process of dying.

Uncertainty or disputation about the prognosis raises the voltage of the fear and potential remorse that is a normal condition of care and support at the end of life. Unilateral decisions and overruling of objections should be avoided when possible, and reinforced by legal or ethical authorities when necessary. An ethics consultant, especially one skilled and experienced in management of end-of-life issues, can be a helpful negotiator and guide.

The transition to palliative support should include the discontinuation of all unnecessary monitoring devices and tubes. Monitors should be turned off allowing families to direct their attention to the patient. Removing the monitor relieves family members from painful suspense and confusion. Removing the endotracheal tube sometimes allows conscious patients to talk to their loved ones, ending a silence forced on them by their treatment. If interventions are seen as masking the natural dying process, removing them should not be troubling. Their absence gives moral clarity to the elemental moments of closure at the end of life, no longer masked by futile contrivance.

Withdrawal of life-sustaining treatment is a process that "merits the same meticulous preparation and expectation of quality that clinicians provide when they perform other procedures to initiate life support" [6]. Families and patients should never feel abandoned during this process and attention should be devoted to communicating that care is not being withdrawn. The family needs to be prepared for what the dying process may look like. Assure them that all energy is now being directed toward the comfort of the patient including sedation as required if signs of suffering are observed.

Easing death, like easing birth, can be one of the most fulfilling contributions one can make to reduce the suffering and enrich the lives of patients and their families. Neglecting this part of the duty to provide appropriate care brings moral anguish to all participants in the peculiar circumstances that have come to surround death in the ICUs of developed countries.

It is helpful to accept the inevitable reality that death is, in Shakespeare's words, a "necessary end" to all mortal life, and to recognize that defying death with technology can sometimes become an unnatural and degrading activity, however well motivated. The withdrawal of life-sustaining treatment, when conducted expertly, is a shared human experience that can be gratifying, although difficult for all concerned.

References

[1] Beauchamp TL, Childress JF. Principles of biomedical ethics. 5th edition. New York: Oxford University Press; 2001.

[2] Rieth KA. How do we withhold or withdraw life-sustaining therapy? Nurs Manage 1999;30:20–5.

[3] Prien T, Van Aken H. Ethical dilemmas in intensive care: can the problem be solved? Curr Opin Anaesthesiol 1999;12:203–6.

[4] Gostin LO. Deciding life and death in the courtroom: from Quinlan to Cruzan, Glucksberg, and Vacco. A brief history and analysis of constitutional protection of the 'right to die'. JAMA 1997;278:1523–8.

[5] Vincent J. Cultural differences in end-of-life care. Crit Care Med 2001;29:N52–5.

[6] Rubenfeld GD, Crawford SW. Principles and practice of withdrawing life-sustaining treatment in the ICU. In: Curtis RJ, Rubenfeld GD, editors. Managing death in the ICU the transition from cure to comfort. New York: Oxford University Press; 2001. p. 127–47.

[7] Gordon M. Whose life is it and who decides? A dilemma in long-term care. Annals of Long Term Care 2004;9:1524.

[8] Seymour JE. Negotiating natural death in intensive care. Soc Sci Med 2000;51:1241–52.

[9] Melltorp G, Nilstun T. The difference between withholding and withdrawing life-sustaining treatment. Intensive Care Med 1997;23:1264–7.

[10] Rosner F. Jewish medical ethics. J Clin Ethics 1995;6: 202–17.

[11] Morrison MF, Demichele SG. How culture and religion affect attitudes toward medical futility. In: Zucker MB, Zucker HD, editors. Medical futility and the evaluation of life-sustaining interventions. New York: Cambridge University Press; 1997. p. 71–82.

[12] Clarfield AM, Gordon M, Markwell H, et al. Ethical issues in end-of-life geriatric care: the approach of three monotheistic religions: Judaism, Catholicism, and Islam. Journal of American Geriatrics Society 2003;51:1149–54.

[13] Weijer C. CPR for patient's in a PVS: futile or acceptable? Can Med Assoc J 1998;158:491–3.

[14] Kunin J. Withholding artificial feeding from the severely demented: merciful or immoral? contrasts between secular and Jewish perspectives. J Med Ethics 2003;29:208–12.

[15] Truog RD, Fackler JC. It is reasonable to reject the diagnosis of brain death. J Clin Ethics 1992;3:80–1.

[16] Kirkland LL. Brain death and the termination of life support: case and analysis. J Clin Ethics 1992;3:78.

[17] Freer JP. Brain death and the termination of life support: case and analysis. J Clin Ethics 1992;3:78.

[18] Vincent J. Forgoing life support in western European intensive care units: the results of an ethical questionnaire. Crit Care Med 1999;27:1626–33.

[19] Levin PD, Sprung CL. Cultural differences at the end of life. Crit Care Med 2003;31:S354–7.

[20] Callahan D. The troubled dream of life: in search of a peaceful death. Washington: Georgetown University Press; 2000.

[21] Cassell EJ. The sorcerer's broom: medicine's rampant technology. Hastings Cent Rep 1993;23:32–9.

[22] Nelson JE, Danis M. End-of-life care in the intensive care unit: where are we now? Crit Care Med 2001; 29(2 Suppl):N2–9.

[23] Wong DT, Gomez M, Mcguire GP, et al. Utilization of intensive care unit days in a Canadian medical-surgical intensive care unit. Crit Care Med 1999;27:1319–24.

[24] Cook D, Rocker G, Marshall J, et al. Withdrawal of

mechanical ventilation in anticipation of death in the intensive care unit. N Engl J Med 2003;349:1123–32.
[25] Prendergast TJ, Puntillo KA. Withdrawal of life support: intensive caring at the end of life. JAMA 2002; 288:2732–40.
[26] Cook DJ, Guyatt GH, Jaeschke R, et al. Determinants in Canadian health care workers of the decision to withdraw life support from the critically ill. Canadian Critical Care Trials Group. JAMA 1995;273:703–8.
[27] Christakis NA, Asch DA. Biases in how physicians choose to withdraw life support. Lancet 1993;342: 642–7.
[28] Fish A, Singer PA, Nancy B. The criminal code and decisions to forgo life-sustaining treatment. Can Med Assoc J 1992;147:637–42.
[29] Lo B. Resolving ethical dilemmas: a guide for clinicians. Baltimore: Williams & Wilkins; 1995.
[30] Luce JM, Alpers A. Legal aspects of withholding and withdrawing life support from critically ill patients in the United States and providing palliative care to them. Am J Respir Care Med 2000;162:2029–32.
[31] Luce JM, Alpers A. End-of-life care: what do the American courts say? Crit Care Med 2001;29:N40–5.
[32] Downie J. Unilateral withholding and withdrawal of life-sustaining treatment: a violation of dignity under the law in Canada. J Palliat Care 2004;20:143–9.
[33] Duffy A, Tam P. Patients, doctors in ethical grey zone. The Ottawa Citizen. April 28, 2005.
[34] American Thoracic Society. Withholding and withdrawing life-sustaining therapy. Am Rev Respir Dis 1991;144:726–31.
[35] Task Force on Ethics of the Society of Critical Care Medicine. Consenus report on the ethics of foregoing life-sustaining treatments in the critically ill. Crit Care Med 1990;18:1435–9.
[36] American Medical Association. E-2.037 Medical futility in end-of-life care. www.ama-assn.org/ama/pub/category/8390.html. Accessed July 25, 2005.
[37] Nolin T, Andersson R. Withdrawal of medical treatment in the ICU: a cohort study of 318 cases during 1994–2000. Acta Anaesthesiol Scand 2003;47:501–7.
[38] Faber-Langendoen KA. Multi-institutional study of care given to patients dying in hospitals. ethical and practice implications. Arch Intern Med 1996;156: 2130–6.
[39] Cook DJ, Guyatt G, Rocker G, et al. Cardiopulmonary resuscitation directives on admission to intensive care unit: an international observational study. Lancet 2001; 358:1941–5.
[40] Fried TR, Bradley EH, Towle VR, et al. Understanding the treatment preferences of seriously ill patients. N Engl J Med 2002;346:1061–6.
[41] Rotondi AJ, Chelluri L, Sirio C, et al. Patients' recollections of stressful experiences while receiving prolonged mechanical ventilation in an intensive care unit. Crit Care Med 2002;30:746–52.
[42] Tonelli MR. Waking the dying: must we always attempt to involve critically ill patients in end-of-life decisions? Chest 2005;127:637–42.
[43] Gottschalk LA, Bechtel RJ, Buchman TG, et al. Computerized content analysis of conversational interactions. Comput Inform Nurs 2003;21:249–58.
[44] Curtis JR, Engelberg RA, Wenrich MD, et al. Missed opportunities during family conferences about end-of-life care in the intensive care unit. Am J Respir Crit Care Med 2005;171:844–9.
[45] Moreau D, Goldgran-Toledano D, Alberti C, et al. Junior versus senior physicians for informing families of intensive care unit patients. Am J Respir Crit Care Med 2004;169:512–7.
[46] Heyland DK, Rocker GM, Dodek PM, et al. Family satisfaction with care in the intensive care unit: results of a multiple center study. Crit Care Med 2002;30: 1413–8.
[47] Pochard F, Azoulay E, Chevret S, et al. Symptoms of anxiety and depression in family members of intensive care unit patients: ethical hypothesis regarding decision-making capacity. Crit Care Med 2001;29: 1893–7.
[48] Happ MB, Kagan SH. Methodological considerations for grounded theory research in critical care settings. Nurs Res 2001;50:188–92.
[49] Gabor JY, Cooper AB, Crombach SA, et al. Contribution of the intensive care unit environment to sleep disruption in mechanically ventilated patients and healthy subjects. Am J Respir Crit Care Med 2003; 167:708–15.
[50] Emanuel EJ, Emanuel LL. Four models of the physician patient relationship. In: Boetzkes E, Waluchow WJ, editors. Readings in health care ethics, vol. 1. 1st edition. Toronto: Broadview Press; 2000. p. 40–9.
[51] Buckman R. How to break bad news: a guide for health care professionals. Baltimore: The Johns Hopkins University Press; 1992.
[52] Coulehan JL, Platt FW, Egener B, et al. "Let me see if I have this right...": words that help build empathy. Ann Intern Med 2001;135:221–7.
[53] Asch DA. The role of critical care nurses in euthanasia and assisted suicide. N Engl J Med 1996;334:1374–9.
[54] Powis J, Etchells E, Martin DK, et al. Can a "good death" be made better? preliminary evaluation of a patient -centered quality improvement strategy for severely ill in-patients. BMC Palliative Care 2004;3: 2–9. Available at: Http://Www.Biomedcentral.Com/1472-684X/3/2. Accessed May 8, 2005.
[55] Patrick DL, Engelberg RA, Curtis JR. Evaluating the quality of dying and death. J Pain Symptom Manage 2001;22:717–26.
[56] Hawryluck LA, Harvey WRC, Lemieux-Charles L, et al. Consensus guidelines on analgesia and sedation in dying intensive care unit patients. BMC Medical Ethics 2002;3:3–12. Available at: Http://Www.Biomedcentral.Com/1472-6939/3/3. Accessed May 8, 2005.
[57] Sneiderman B, Deutscher R. Dr. Nancy Morrison and her dying patient: a case of medical necessity. Health Law J 2002;10:1–30.
[58] Truog RD, Cist AF, Brackett SE, et al. Recommen-

dations for end-of-life care in the intensive care unit: the Ethics Committee of the Society of Critical Care Medicine. Crit Care Med 2001;29:2332–48.

[59] Riker RR, Fraser GL, Rohr WB, et al. Neuromuscular blockade at the end of life. N Engl J Med 2000;342: 1921–2.

[60] Johnson N, Cook D, Giacomini M, et al. Towards a "good" death: end-of-life narratives constructed in an intensive care unit. Cult Med Psychiatry 2000;24:275.

[61] Goold SD, Williams B, Arnold RM. Conflicts regarding decisions to limit treatment: a differential diagnosis. JAMA 2000;283:909–14.

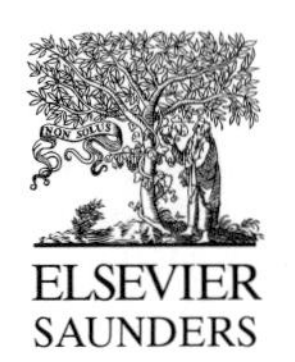
ELSEVIER
SAUNDERS

Thorac Surg Clin 15 (2005) 481 – 491

THORACIC
SURGERY
CLINICS

Postoperative Futile Care: Stopping the Train When the Family Says "Keep Going"

K. Francis Lee, MD, MPH, FACS

Department of Surgery, Baystate Medical Center, Tufts University School of Medicine, Springfield, MA 01199, USA

Withdrawal of life-support has become a common mode of death in ICUs across the country. In 1998, a national survey of 131 ICUs from 38 states revealed that 70% of the ICU deaths occurred by withdrawal or withholding of support, including cardiopulmonary resuscitation [1]. Medically appropriate end-of-life care decisions are often fraught with conflict among decision-makers. Physicians, nurses, and the family experience conflict in most ICU cases, and most of them involve the issue of life-sustaining treatments [2]. In most cases, the care providers prefer aggressive treatment more than the family does. In 24% of the time, however, it is the family-surrogate who desires aggressive treatments over the care providers' reservations [1]. Fortunately, the conflict usually is resolved without undue consequences, and very few patients actually receive futile care for any significant period. Narrowly defined, futile treatments reportedly account for only 2% to 4% of total ICU bed use [3,4].

Beyond the economic costs, however, the family's demand for seemingly futile medical care creates an enormous emotional toll for care providers. Weighed against the principle of patient autonomy is the less recognized but equally important concept of professional conscience and integrity. When both requirements are unsatisfied, risk of dissatisfactory medical care, medicolegal liability, and eventually professional burnout arises. The editor has posed the question: How does the surgeon "stop the train" when the family says "keep going"? This article reviews the definition of "futile" care, the limits of physician autonomy vis-à-vis that of patient autonomy, the legal ramifications and precedents of futile care, and recommendations for a surgeon.

Definition of futile care

The Society of Critical Care Medicine's Ethics Committee published a consensus statement in which the following definitions of medically futile treatments are offered

> Since these conflicts are typically about differences in *values* rather than disagreements about *facts*, clinicians should be very cautious about labeling these therapeutic options as futile. Seen in this context, ("futile") treatments may be classified into four categories: a) treatments that have no beneficial physiologic effect; b) treatments that are extremely unlikely to be beneficial; c) treatments that have beneficial effect but are extremely costly; d) treatments that are of uncertain or controversial benefit.
>
> Treatments that fall into the first category, i.e., those treatments that offer no physiologic benefit to the patient, should be labeled as *futile*. Treatments that fall into the other three categories may be considered *inappropriate and hence inadvisable*, but should not be labeled futile [5].

According to their strict definition, a truly "futile" care is tantamount to a therapy that does not have an indication for use because a benefit based on medical science is absent. Such a therapy should not be offered or provided, and it should not create a

E-mail address: francis.lee@bhs.org

1547-4127/05/$ – see front matter
doi:10.1016/j.thorsurg.2005.06.005

controversy. For "inappropriate and inadvisable" therapy, however, the difficulty lies in attempts to define futility based on any quantitative probability of benefit. Physicians disagree greatly on the definition of futility based on success rate [6]. When asked about the probability of treatment success selected as a cutoff defining futility, 15% of the physicians chose 11% to 25% chance of success as a cutoff, whereas 35% chose 1% to 5% as the cutoff for futility [7]. Even the most conservative criteria of less than 1% engendered critiques and counterarguments in the literature [8].

Prognostication is difficult on a case-by-case basis, whether the estimation is calculated by established prediction models [5] or the physician's clinical judgment. The case of Baby Ryan Nguyen is illustrative. In the case of a premature neonate with brain damage, intestinal obstruction, and renal failure, two hospitals refused to continue to provide dialysis, citing as reason "no likelihood of a good outcome" and "universally fatal" prognosis [9]. The family obtained a temporary court order to force dialysis treatment until the full trial, but the case never went to court because they located a facility willing to provide the necessary treatment [9]. Apparently, according to the physicians' critics, the baby's condition improved, and "Ryan lived four years, a happy if sickly child who gave high-fives and was the delight of his parents' hearts" [10].

Central to the criticism of a quantitative definition of futility is a distrust of physicians' paternalistic assessment of what constitutes an unreasonable hope for success, or an unacceptable quality of life. Arguably, families ought to have the option to continue treatment if it provides the slightest glimmer of hope [11]. Attempts to define futility based on medical conditions of very poor prognosis and quality of life, such as terminal cancer, irreversible coma, or advanced cirrhosis, may be criticized for insensitivity and neglect of the patient's or surrogate's values. Presently, the pendulum of control over quality-of-life judgment has swung to patient and surrogate, not to the medical professional. The surgeon's certainty of poor outcome based on prognosis or quality of life alone is not sufficient to conclude that a treatment is futile for all parties involved.

Ultimately, a precise definition for medical futility is impossible. A qualified definition of medical futility (ie, inappropriate and inadvisable therapy) must account for both the probability of therapeutic benefit and the patient's and surrogate's beliefs and values as evinced by their expression of preferences and goals of treatment. The American Medical Association Council on Ethical and Judicial Affairs commented, futility "cannot be meaningfully defined" [12]. Most surgeons, however, would concur with Halevy's comment: "we certainly know it when we see it" [13].

Anatomy of Conflict

In most postoperative futility cases facing the thoracic surgeon, the patient is incapacitated and the decision-maker is a surrogate appointed by a health care proxy or next-of-kin family member. When the surrogate rejects the recommendation for withdrawal of support, the surgeon should consider three reasons for the refusal: (1) inadequate communication skills, (2) emotional problems, and (3) values misalignment. When the patient's prognosis is poor, the surgeon may feel compelled to use euphemisms to protect the family from emotional trauma. A hopeless prognosis, however, is better communicated using clear words. For example, "Your father is dying and has no hope of recovery." Softening the blow with equivocal expressions only contributes to lingering hope and indecision of the family. Sometimes the surrogate needs to hear, "death," "no hope," "impossible," clearly and repetitively to be released from false hope to reach a realistic expectation of terminal outcome. This release begins the next phase of bereavement. The surgeon must refrain from technical terminologies, such as "functional status," "median survival," "sepsis," "pressors," which confound rather than clarify the surrogate's understanding. Even a highly educated family member experiences reduction in their intellectual reasoning capacity during an acute illness and medical crisis. The surgeon should remember to use simple language that even a person with a minimal education may comprehend.

In 1995, Tulsky and coworkers [14] audiotaped interviews of medical residents and surrogates discussing ICU do-not-resuscitate (DNR) orders. The residents dominated the interviews by talking 75% of the time and listening very little. The interviews lasted a median of 10 minutes, and few questions were asked of the surrogates. When the surrogates resist withdrawal of support in futile situations, the surgeon should use open-ended questions to determine the reasons for the refusal. Open-ended questions may trigger a response that guides further exploration:

- Tell me your understanding of your wife's medical condition.
- What do you think is happening to your husband?

- What would your father have wanted in this condition?
- What does withdrawing support (pulling the tube) mean to you?

Responses may include the following:

Perhaps the cause may be a gap in comprehension of the dire clinical situation: "My wife has been sick in the ICU before, and she has pulled through and surprised us; I expect she'll do it again."

Perhaps the cause may be one of distrust and confusion: "Since the surgery and the complications, we have not gotten any straight answers, and we don't know what to believe any more."

Perhaps fear of abandonment and suffering: "I don't want to see her suffer and struggle for breath if you pull the tube."

Perhaps guilt: "I know what I have to do, but I'm not sure if I can live with myself for the rest of my life if I let you pull the tube on him."

Perhaps familial strife: "I'm with you on withdrawing support, but my brother doesn't want it to happen that way; I have to have his support, or else I can't let you do it. He's my brother; I don't want to hurt him."

Perhaps personal values: "My father has always lived his life with gusto; he's a fighter, and I know he would have fought right to the end for us."

Perhaps cultural bias and suspicion: "You're just not going to pull the plug on him and give up (like you did to all my people before)."

Perhaps religious values: "We believe she is in God's hands, and He will pull her through; nobody should be making decisions for God."

Perhaps profound emotional deadlock: "This is my boy—you're just not going to take him away from me."

It takes time to overcome these barriers. The surgeon should prepare for a protracted process of query, discovery, and negotiation of a multitude of complex barriers. Any wish for a quick resolution only leads to frustration and emotional drain on the caregivers' part, and possibly an unhealthy surgeon-surrogate relationship.

Repetitive reinforcement of the realistic understanding of the hopeless nature of the case addresses unrealistic comprehension of the clinical situation. An in-depth discussion of the use of analgesia and anxiolytics alleviates the fear of the patient suffering, whereas assurance of aggressive palliative care following withdrawal of ventilatory support may counter the fear of abandonment. To break the barriers of family gridlock, guilt, and personal feelings, it is important to guide the surrogate to focus on the patient's wishes, not those of the surrogate or other family members. In extreme cases, it may be helpful to point out clearly and firmly that the legal responsibility of a health care proxy or a surrogate is to implement only the patient's wishes not those of others. The significance of cultural or religious barriers should not be underestimated. Certain ethnicities, such as African Americans, have a traumatic history of mistreatment from the medical community. Consistent with some African Americans' concerns about health care discrimination, a recent report on Medicare beneficiaries observed wide disparities in mortality and selected medical-surgical services between blacks and whites [15]. It is best to address such concerns by demonstrating that the care level has been appropriately intensive and after withdrawal of support, ICU care continues with equally aggressive palliative care. Surgeons should not have the delusion that these discussions are easy or resolved in one meeting. Multiple family conferences with repetitive reinforcements and reassurances may be necessary. One caveat is that even within a culture or religion, different beliefs prevail; the surgeon should not make broad assumptions that might prove erroneous [16]. Refusal to withdraw support often may arise from specific individual factors, not from cultural or religious influences. In some cases, involving a cultural expert or a religious representative may be helpful.

Additionally, one must be aware of family-surrogates with a strong "sanctity-of-life" belief system. As professionals in the present "divided" America, surgeons should not underestimate the depth of religious convictions. Many believe it is morally wrong to end a patient's life intentionally or to allow a patient's life to end without available interventions [17]. Any discussion invoking quality or the relative value of existence may be unacceptable to the sanctity-of-life world view. At the core lies the conflict of values between the absolute, religious convictions about human life in any form vis-à-vis the relativist approach to the medical futility debate exercised by most physicians. Trivialization of the sanctity-of-life beliefs, insensitivity, or disrespect for such believers only leads to an impasse between the family-surrogate and surgeon [17]. Some of the most publicized legal cases of medical futility have involved surrogate decision-makers who have asserted a religious, sanctity-of-life justification for continued life-supportive measures: *Wanglie* [18], *Baby K* [19], and *Schiavo* [20].

When surgeons encounter a roadblock based on a surrogate's values that differ from theirs, it is critical to shift from the mental framework of "obtain-a-consent" to that of "negotiate-a-solution." First, discover and understand the surrogate's values, preferences, and goals of treatment for the patient. Surprisingly, few clinicians spend adequate time to understand fully the surrogate's perspective, and the most common cause of negotiation failure is the physicians' lack of understanding [21]. The moral integrity of all parties deserves respect and it should not be violated. Openly state the differences of value if they exist, and then begin to address them in a problem-solving manner, not as a battle over moral conflicts. Key to successful negotiation is continuously to set aside the nonessential differences, while striving to find one or two important points on which to build solutions. For example, when a Muslim surrogate refuses withdrawal of ventilator support based on his religion's rejection of brain death, an agreement can still be reached on the therapeutic goal of avoiding needless suffering or preventing heroic means of prolonging poor quality of life, neither of which Islam supports [22]. Negotiation is further aided by the caregivers' respectful attention to the patient's and surrogate's values, which for Muslims are their ritualistic needs of daily prayers; fastidious care of bodily discharges (and wounds); and gender-specific modesty [22].

In the end, when most physician-surrogate conflicts resolve over time in response to new clinical developments, as they do in most cases, the resolution occurs more as a result of established trust, respect, and mutual understanding of good will, rather than from any argumentative sway or intellectual breakthrough. In this regard, the adage "Surgeon, know thy self" becomes paramount. Surgeons should evaluate their own feelings vis-à-vis that of the surrogate. After a difficult physician-surrogate conference, the surgeon's feelings of anger (against challenge of authority), outrage (toward the surrogate), guilt (over the development of complications), or fear (of liability) must be acknowledged and addressed by the surgeon alone and "put to bed" before any further discussion with the surrogate continues.

The more surgeons become emotionally neutral, other than maintaining sympathy and compassion, the more they can constructively explore the surrogate's emotions. Caring for the surrogate's emotional experience is beneficial to negotiation. In a study of families who have had a member in the ICU withdrawn from support [23], the caregivers' behaviors including nonverbal communications greatly affected the burden of their decision-making. The care providers' understanding of the families' unmet emotional needs proved helpful to the decision-making process. In the interviews, the families recommended to the care providers active communication of critical information in a timely and coordinated manner; assistance with resolving family conflicts; understanding and accommodating their grief and bereavement; and, establishing advance directives with the patients themselves before surgery [23].

Patient's (surrogate's) autonomy versus surgeon's professional integrity

Despite the care providers' assiduous efforts to resolve a conflict, they sometimes encounter a roadblock of religious and personal values more formidable than any negotiating skills. In rare cases, conflict resolution is elusive and unreachable. The following statements by Helga Wanglie's family [18] demonstrate, for example, an unflinching, resolute stance by the surrogates: "Mother (patient)...said that if anything happened to her, she wouldn't want her life prematurely shortened if she wasn't able to take care of herself" [24]. The patient's husband commented, "...only God can take life and...doctors should not play God" [25]. With each passing day of apparent futile care, the caregivers begin to suffer from a gnawing sense of violating their own professional conscience and integrity. In such a case, the issue of "patient versus physician autonomy" looms large. Eventually, the question emerges, "Who is in charge"? Is it conscionable, ethically defensible, or legally safe for the surgeon to withdraw support unilaterally over the surrogate's objections?

For the surrogate and the family, the right to privacy and self-determination is not only supported by today's cultural ethos, but it is also a Constitutional principle supported by the courts [26]. The lesser known concept of professional conscience dealing with matters of medical futility is derived historically from the traditions of Hippocrates and various religions. According to Hippocrates, "to attempt futile treatment is to display an ignorance that is allied with madness" [27]. Jewish rabbinical teachings prescribe withholding treatments in the state of gesisah within 72 hours of death [28,29]. Although a surprising papal statement in 2004 supported the use of artificial nutrition and hydration in persistent vegetative state and caused a great deal of confusion among Catholic bioethicists [30], a long-established Catholic ethical tradition has always distinguished between "ordinary or proportionate treatment" and "extraordinary or disproportionate treatment" [31], and has upheld to the modern times by Vatican declarations and other papal statements the notion of withholding life-sustaining treatments that are "disproportionate" or "burdensome." Modern United States public policy statements also support the concept of medical futility, such as from the President's Commission for the Study of Ethical Problems in Medicine and Biomedical and Behavioral Research [32].

Surgeons' opposition to futile treatment is arguably based on three of the four basic ethical principles: (1) beneficence: prevent or remove the patient's unnecessary suffering from hopeless medical condition; (2) nonmaleficence: avoid infliction of harm (inclusive of invasive treatments without likelihood of benefit); and (3) distributive justice: allocate resources equitably among patients. The issue of health care resource allocation as it relates to medical futility is not addressed in this article. Although pertinent as a societal and health care system issue, the debate surrounding distributive justice is not a common cause of physician-patient conflict over end-of-life care decisions. One can even extend the fourth principle of autonomy to cover their right to practice free from coercion to provide treatment against their will. All these ethical considerations for surgeons' professional integrity can be countered, however, by the argument of the patient's right to self-determination. Based on ethical considerations alone, the answer to the question "who is in charge" remains equivocal and indeterminate.

When practical or ethical considerations fall short of a convincing solution, surgeons may look for legal answers, preferably a court decision in favor of their cause. Surgeons hoping that the courtroom provides an end to a medical futility impasse, however, may be disappointed. No clear, consistent jurisprudence on medical futility exists. A review of common law cases in the past three decades suggests that the courts have decided in favor of both sides with the ultimate judgment depending on the highly fact-specific context of individual cases as much as any relevant legal doctrine in the jurisdiction.

Patient autonomy has been well-tested in such landmark cases as *Karen Quinlan* [26] and *Nancy Cruzan* [33], and codified in federal legislation, the Patient Self-Determination Act of 1990 [34]. The principle of physician's professional integrity, however, has also received legal attention [35–38]. In *Superintendent of Belchertown v Saikewicz*, the Supreme Judicial Court of Massachusetts expressed "maintaining the ethical integrity of the medical profession" as one of the key state interests to be considered by the court in rendering its decision [35]. A few common law cases also have upheld the physician's right to refuse providing care contrary to professional conscience [36–38].

State statutes have specifically referred to physician autonomy in medically futile cases. A section of the Virginia Health Care Decisions Act under the subheading "Medically unnecessary treatment not required" was amended specifically to state "Nothing in this article shall be construed to require a physician to prescribe or render medical treatment to a patient that the physician determines to be medically or ethically inappropriate" [39]. In 1993, the Maryland Health Care Decisions Act also codified the physician's right to refuse treatments determined to be "ethically inappropriate" or "medically ineffective" [40]. Texas and California have statutes outlining processes by which a physician may withhold treatment against the wishes of patient-surrogates [41,42]. California statutes further specify the health care provider's rights to "decline for reasons of conscience or institutional policy," or to "decline to comply with an instruction or decision that requires the provision of care which would be medically ineffective or contrary to generally accepted health-care standards" [43].

Furthermore, when legal action is brought by the surrogates following the death of the patient, some legal precedents seem to validate the physician's right to unilaterally withdraw life-sustaining treatments. Charges of infliction of emotional suffering, abandonment, or intentional battery have not been upheld.

- In *Gilgunn v Massachusetts General Hospital* (1995) [44], a daughter of a 72-year-old woman with multiorgan system failure and severe neurologic devastation sued the hospital for neglect and infliction of emotional suffering. She asserted that the hospital failed to treat her mother adequately with cardiopulmonary resuscitation and let her die with a DNR order without her consent. The jury quickly found in favor of the physicians and the hospital, reasoning no breach of care to the patient occurred. This case was believed to herald a new trend in the jurisprudence of medical futility end-of-life decision-making in favor of the physicians and the hospitals.
- In *Bryan v Rectors and Visitors of the University of Virginia* (1996) [45], a terminally ill woman was transferred and admitted to the ICU with respiratory failure. The physicians entered a

DNR order against the family's wishes and 12 days later the patient had a heart attack and died without any resuscitation efforts. The court rejected the family's claim of abandonment of care and ruled in favor of the physicians and the hospital.

- In *Causey v St. Francis Medical Center* (1998) [46], the hospital and physician withdrew life-sustaining care from a 31-year-old woman with quadriplegia, end-stage renal failure, and persistent vegetative state over the family's objections. The family initially filed a suit alleging treatment without consent and an intentional battery-based tort causing the patient's death. The district court dismissed the suit as premature because withdrawal of support constituted a medical procedure covered under the Medical Malpractice Act. The physician was entitled to withhold care as long as it was within standards of medical care. The family appealed, but the appellate court agreed that it was not an intentional battery, but rather a medical procedure that should have been submitted for medical review before the lawsuit [46].

In these rulings, the courts placed limits on physicians' legal obligation to provide care deemed futile and outside standard of care. A cursory look might suggest that a surgeon enjoys strong legal rights to deny care to a medically futile case whenever desired without the surrogate's consent. A careful analysis, however, cautions against such an interpretation. In *Gilgunn*, for example, the jury only spent 2 hours to find no liability for the physicians, using their own definition of futile treatment as that which does not provide cure. The jury failed to acknowledge a different definition of futility based on quality of life even if cure is possible. Futility as narrowly defined by physicians without considering the patient's or the surrogate's values for quality or meaning of life is fraught with legal problems, especially from the viewpoint of disability laws [47]. It has been pointed out that *Gilgunn* was only a lower court decision; its judicial weight as precedence is limited [48]. Daar [49] has commented that no court has ever found the integrity of the medical profession compelling enough to serve as the sole basis for ignoring the patient's right of self-determination, or even to suggest that physician integrity and patient autonomy deserve equal weight.

In *Bryan*, the plaintiffs asserted that abandonment was in the framework of the Emergency Medical Treatment and Labor Act (EMTALA). In a previous case involving the EMTALA [50], the appellate court *In re Baby K* had ruled that the federal law bound the physicians in the emergency department to provide acute respiratory care to the anencephalic baby no matter how futile the treatments seemed to the care providers. In *Bryan,* the court narrowly defined EMTALA as pertaining to emergency care only, and ruled that the law did not apply to patients in the ICU after hospital admission for ongoing care. The case was more of a judgment that attempted to limit the scope of EMTALA, reversing its previous controversial decision in *Baby K*, than it was of expanding the physicians' professional autonomy.

Some state statutes also limit the physician's ability to act unilaterally and provide language to ensure that the patient's or the surrogate's decision is respected. The Virginia Act explains, "...if the physician's determination is contrary to the terms of an advance directive of a qualified patient or the treatment decision of a person designated to make the decision . . ., the physician shall make a reasonable effort to inform the patient or the patient's designated decision-maker of such determination and the reasons for the determination" [39]. Under Maryland law, a physician may not take any medical action when the patient or surrogate has "expressed disagreement with the action" [40]. Both statutes require the physician to offer an opportunity for transfer of the patient to another physician or medical facility. The Virginia Act exhorts, "The physician shall provide the patient or his authorized decision-maker a reasonable time of not less than fourteen days to affect such transfer. During this period, the physician shall continue to provide any life-sustaining care to the patient which is reasonably available to such physician, as requested by the patient or his designated decision-maker" [39]. In Texas, a similar statutory requirement exists for transfer of care [41].

"Transfer of care" is used as a legal device to ensure the physician's professional rights are balanced against those of the patient-surrogates. This legislative safeguard has been exercised several times. Even when the physician's right to deny futile treatments was upheld, the courts have required them to offer transfer of care to the patient-surrogates [36–38]. In some cases, the court has only required the physician to offer the opportunity but did not require that the physician personally arrange the transfer. That responsibility was left to the patient's surrogate and the family [36]. In other instances, the court has specifically ordered the institution, not the physician, directly to assist the patient's transfer to a suitable facility [38,51]. Based on these legal precedents, any surgeon who is contemplating withdrawal of support over the surrogate's objection should offer a transfer of care to another physician or facility before any unilateral action is contemplated. A reasonable effort to transfer the patient should be documented in the medical records.

In reality, transfer of care is difficult in a medical futility case when ethical and legal complexities raise the possibility of legal liability. To have another physician or institution accept the dying patient is a difficult prospect. In *In re Wanglie*, for example, no physician emerged to take over the care of the patient [18]. It is precisely the failure of transfer of care that typically forces either the care provider or the surrogate to resort to legal action [18,36,52].

On several occasions, physicians have approached the courts to rule on the question, "Who is in charge"? This action directly challenges the surrogate's decision-making. While the patient is still alive, the courts are loathe to take responsibility for overtly invalidating the surrogate's decision that may lead to the patient's death. They have been unwilling to comply with the hospital's request to challenge or negate the surrogate's right to decide for the patient. Since the *Karen Quinlan* ruling in 1976, courts frequently have rejected a challenge to surrogacy [53].

- *In re Wanglie* (1991) [18], the physicians sought to terminate the mechanical ventilation of an 85-year-old woman in persistent vegetative state, because it was "inappropriate medical treatment" and "no longer serving the patient's personal best interest." The patient's husband, however, insisted on continued respiratory support. The court struck down the hospital's request for a conservator who would determine the patient's "best interest," reasoning that the patient's husband of 53 years was the best proxy under the circumstances to decide for the patient.
- *In re Jane Doe* (1992) [54], the mother agreed to a DNR order for her 13-year-old daughter with a degenerative neurologic disease, but the father did not agree. The trial court ruled that both parents must agree for the hospital to enter a DNR order. On appeal to the Supreme Court of Georgia, it was affirmed that the agreement of both parents was indeed required for a DNR order, thereby disallowing "de-escalation" of treatment as requested by the hospital.
- *In re Baby K* (1993) [19], the hospital pleaded to the court that providing repeated ventilatory respiratory care to an anencephalic baby in the emergency department is medically inappropriate. The court ruled, however, that anencephaly is a disability covered under the Americans with Disabilities Act of 1990; denial of treatment is prohibited under the law [17,19]. When the hospital appealed, the US Court of Appeals for the Fourth Circuit upheld the lower court's decision by invoking the EMTALA to impose on the hospital a duty to treat under the federal law [50]. In this case, two federal legislations were cited to uphold the surrogate's decision for continued treatment.
- Barbara Howe (1998–current) [55], is a 79-year-old woman with advanced amyotrophic lateral sclerosis and progressive cerebral dysfunction. In a persistent vegetative state, she has been dependent on a mechanical ventilator for over 5 years. The physicians and the hospital have asked the Massachusetts Probate and Family Court to intervene in their dispute with the patient's daughter who demanded continued aggressive care. The judge ruled insufficient cause to overturn the daughter as her mother's health care proxy, disallowing the physicians to withdraw support.

To be sure, courts have appointed independent guardians in cases where quarreling parents of minors or parents with "specific incompetence" were unable to agree about appropriate care [56,57]. Nevertheless, the courts' reluctance to overturn the rights of legal surrogates is nowhere demonstrated more vividly than in the recent case of *Theresa Schiavo*. Theresa Schiavo was a 41-year-old woman in persistent vegetative state following anoxic brain injury from cardiac arrest 14 years ago. Her husband was the judicially appointed guardian. His right and request for removal of feeding tube was repeatedly upheld by various Florida courts. The courts found the husband's depiction of the patient's prior verbal wishes as "clear and convincing" evidence that she would choose to forego additional care in the circumstances. Despite enormous political pressure from the legislative and the executive branches of the state and the federal government, the Florida 2nd District Court of Appeals, the Florida Supreme Court, and the US Supreme Court repeatedly denied the patient's parents' motions to transfer the guardianship or to stay the order to remove the feeding tube [20]. On March 18, 2005, Mrs. Schiavo's feeding tube was removed according to the guardian's instruction to carry out the patient's "clear and convincing" wish, and the patient passed away 13 days later [58].

Given the political and legislative clashes surrounding the Schiavo case, it is difficult to imagine that any court would casually transfer the surrogacy in a medical futility debate. Nor would they be expected to force a medical treatment against the surrogate's wishes. A surgeon or a hospital approaching the court with the purpose of challenging the surrogate's competence or "best interest" decision-making should expect many legal challenges. Ultimately, the surgeon must question whether anything can be gained by seeking legal intervention. As difficult as it may seem, some surgeons might adhere to their professional conscience and withdraw life-sustaining treatments over the surrogate's objections. They then must be willing to accept the risk of legal action as in *Gilgunn*, *Bryan*, and *Causey*. For others, where the risks may outweigh their need for professional autonomy, they might comply with the surrogate's wishes and continue the life-sustaining treatments.

Stopping the train

How does a surgeon who desires to withdraw life-sustaining care in a futile postoperative condition minimize the risks of subsequent legal action and liability? The following two principles of action are offered. First, the surgeon should display utmost professionalism based on compassion, openness, and attention to the clinical needs of both the patient and the family. Some legal experts argue that during end-of-life care decisions on insensate patients, protection of the family becomes the physician's primary obligation [48]. The Institute of Medicine has commented in *When Children Die*, "One goal of palliative and end-of-life care is to minimize avoidable conflicts related to poor communication, cultural misunderstandings, deficient clinical care, and approaches to decision making that fail to assure families that they and the health care team are doing their best for the child" [59]. Similar principles apply to the care of an adult patient's family and surrogate. When families looked back 1 year after discussing withdrawal of support in the ICU, about half of them recalled having conflicts, mostly with the medical staff [60]. The most recurring themes were communication problems and "unprofessional/disrespectful behavior by the doctors and nurses." These two elements predispose a physician to malpractice litigation.

When a surgeon's futility decision becomes a cause of subsequent legal action, the record should reflect professional behavior beyond reproach. When faced with a legal impasse, the court recognizes that there must be a winner and a loser in the adversarial contest, and it must decide which party must be made to suffer [49]. In such a case, a legal defense of professional integrity (the cornerstone of the physician's argument in futility debates) rings hollow if the court documents show a pattern of professional behavior that has been intentionally insensitive and inhumane to the patient and family. When the opposing parties negotiated an agreement to withdraw support from Barbara Howe by June 2005, each party equally acknowledged the other's role. The hospital stated, "...the family has acted out of love and concern for their mother" while the family replied "...the hospital acted with similar concern for (their) patient and that Barbara would not have received better care anywhere else" [61]. The courts seize opportunities to comment on the physician's conduct whenever it is salient. During one case, the California Court of Appeal commended the physician for behaving "according to the highest standards of the medical profession" as it upheld his right to abandon long-term care of an unreasonable patient [36]. Courts made similar comments in the Schiavo litigation [20].

Surgeons should not engage in a unilateral withdrawal of care as isolated, individual practitioners. Decisions to withdraw care should be deliberated in an open, fair process involving the hospital resources for conflict resolution and risk management. A second independent surgeon with a similar level of expertise should be obtained as a consultant to document an objective assessment that corroborates or dissents from the initial clinical recommendation. The hospital ethics committee involvement is a necessary step, considering the literature support for its role and benefit in futility conflicts [62–64]. Legal experts affirm consultations from the ethics committee as an important procedural step when viewed retrospectively [65]. The courts often remark on the ethics committee's deliberations in their own opinions. In Texas, an ethics committee evaluation is required before the physician or the hospital is allowed to withdraw support against the wishes of the surrogate [41].

Because of the failure to agree on the definition or the solution to futility, recent emphasis has been placed on a fair and open process to which all parties can adhere [63]. Institutions should establish a process for determining futile conditions [3,11,13]. Preferably, the process should include clear communication; negotiation; and if appropriate, impartial arbitration [66]. The process could also be a multi-institutional policy of regional health care providers [13]. In turn, institutional policies should rely on published statements and policies of major professional organizations [5,67–69]. It has been postulated that an institutional policy might shift the burden of legal challenge from the physicians to the patient's family [70]. Courts will take into account whether the denial of treatment followed good procedural standards [65], and whether they have shown "extreme deference to pre-existing policies that govern the provision or denial of medical care" [70]. A California statute has delineated health care providers' right to decline treatment "for reasons of conscience or institutional policy" [43], and a Texas law specifically describes the steps required for the physician to withhold life-sustaining treatments over the objections of the surrogate [41].

The fair and open process must respect the integrity of the patient (or the surrogate), the physician, and the institution alike. The Council on Ethical and Judicial Affairs of American Medical Association has proposed a fair process in futility cases that incorporates major principles outlined previously [63]. Sequential steps recommended in the process are

1. Deliberate prior values (if disagreed, offer transfer of care).
2. If values are aligned, pursue joint decision-making using outcomes data and value judgments.
3. If unresolved, involve consultants.
4. If unresolved, involve ethics committee.
5. If unresolved, attempt to transfer within institution.
6. If not possible, attempt to transfer to another institution.
7. If not possible, cease futile intervention.

For the last step, the authors reasoned that if a physician or an institution cannot be found to accept the patient's wishes, it may be because "the request is considered offensive to medical ethics and professional standards in the eyes of a majority of the health care profession." Hence, the authors rationalized that in such circumstances, it is appropriate to cease further futile intervention, but they acknowledged "the legal ramifications of this course of action are uncertain" [63].

This comment is foreboding, especially in the post-Schiavo cultural milieu. Although the jurisprudence on the issues of medical futility is fragile and constantly changing, the Schiavo case has unleashed a remarkable torrent of support from those with strong sanctity-of-life religious convictions. Whether the Schiavo case represents a new political-legislative-judicial trend or just an isolated cultural event remains to be seen. It has renewed efforts to apply the disability laws to the futility cases, however, attempting to define patients with severe neurologic deficit as "disabled persons" whose rights have been grounded as a legal principle in the United States courts. In the context of a range of neurologic deficits and ill-defined distinction between "disability" and "futility," the current public debate resembles the dispute about when life begins. In the Florida Senate, a bill has been introduced, evocatively entitled Starvation and Dehydration of Persons with Disabilities Prevention Act [20]. Similar bills have been introduced in other states. It is possible that surgeons will be held to a different set of state laws in the coming decades from those of the past. It is then anticipated that the conflict at the bedside over medical futility will increase, not decrease, in coming years. It remains to be seen how the courts will evolve with the shifting cultural and political landscape of the "red-blue" America.

Summary

All surgeons must take risks when providing medical care. No guarantees of protection from a lawsuit exist in any guise. Concerning postoperative futile care, the stakes are high when withdrawal of support seems to be indicated but the surrogate believes in sanctity-of-life and demands continued aggressive care. Open-ended questions posed to the family may initiate a dialog that help the surgeon understand their values and negotiate a resolution. Other preventive measures can also reduce the chance of conflict and potential liability.

"Do what's right" is a proverbial motto in surgical training and clinical practice. To some surgeons, it may be to honor the wishes of the family surrogate. To others, the right thing may be to withdraw care in the best interest of the patient. If so, "do what's right" is not just to "stop the train." It also consists of a range of clinical activities, including effective communication, emotional care, and pursuing a fair and open negotiation process established by the institution. Properly conducted, "stopping the train" should incur no greater risk for professional liability than any other challenging procedure that surgeons perform. Withdrawal of futile care should be considered as a procedure, and as such, the skills to deliver it should be mastered like any other.

Acknowledgments

The author acknowledges the invaluable support and help of Barbara A. Noah, JD, in researching the pertinent legal material.

References

[1] Prendergast TJ, Claessens MT, Luce JM. A national survey of end-of-life care for critically ill patients. Am J Respir Crit Care Med 1998;158(4):1163–7.

[2] Breen CM, Abernethy AP, Abbott KH, et al. Conflict associated with decisions to limit life-sustaining treatment in intensive care units. J Gen Intern Med 2001; 16:283–9.

[3] Halevy A, Neal RC, Brody BA. The low frequency of futility in as adult intensive care unit setting. Arch Intern Med 1996;156:100–4.

[4] Sachdeva RC, Jefferson LS, Coss-Bu J, et al. Resource consumption and the extent of futile care among patients in a pediatric intensive care unit setting. J Pediatr 1996;128:742–7.

[5] The Ethics Committee of the Society of Critical Care of Medicine. Consensus statement of the Society of Critical Care Medicine's Ethics Committee regarding futile and other possibly inadvisable treatments. Crit Care Med 1997;25:887–91.

[6] Lantos JD, Singer PA, Walker RM, et al. The illusion of futility in clinical practice. Am J Med 1989;87: 81–4.

[7] McCrary SV, Swanson JW, Youngner SJ, et al. Physicians' quantitative assessments of medical futility. J Clin Ethics 1994;5:100–4.

[8] Schneiderman LJ, Jecker NS, Jonsen AR. Medical futility: response to critiques. Ann Intern Med 1996; 125:669–74.

[9] Capron AM. Baby Ryan and virtual futility. Hastings Cent Rep 1995;(Mar–Apr):20.

[10] Smith W. Can hospitals have the right to pull your plug? San Francisco Chronicle December 2, 2001. Available: Prolife Infonet News Summary, http://www.priestsforlife.org/news/infonet/infonet01-12-03.htm. [Accessed on March 20, 2005.]

[11] Cantor MD, Braddock CH, Derse AR, et al. Do-Not-Resuscitate orders and medical futility. Arch Intern Med 2003;163:2689–94.

[12] Council on Ethical and Judicial Affairs, American Medical Association. *Code of Medical Ethics*. Chicago, Il: American Medical Association; 1994.

[13] Halevy A, Brody BA. a Multi-institution collaborative policy on medical futility. JAMA 1996;276:571–4.

[14] Tulsky JA, Chesney MA, Lo B. How do medical residents discuss resuscitation with patients? J Gen Intern Med 1995;10:436–42.

[15] Gornick ME, Eggers PW, Reilly TW, et al. Effects of race and income on mortality and use of services among Medicare beneficiaries. NEJM 1996;335:791–9.

[16] Hern HE, Koenig BA, Moore LJ, et al. The difference that culture can make in end-of-life decisionmaking. Camb Q Healthc Ethics 1998;7:27–40.

[17] Post SG. Baby K: Medical futility and the free exercise of religion. J Law Med Ethics 1995;23:20–6.

[18] *In re* Wanglie, No. PX-91–283 (Minn. Dist. Ct. 1991).

[19] *In re Baby K*, 832 F. Supp. 1022 (E.D. Va 1993).

[20] Noah BA. Politicizing the End of Life: Lessons from the Schiavo Controversy. Univ Miami Law Rev 2004; 59:107–34.

[21] Dunn PM, Levinson W. Discussing futility with patients and families. J Gen Intern Med 1996;11:689–93.

[22] Sarhill N, LeGrand S, Islambouli M, et al. The terminally ill Muslim: Death and dying from the Muslim perspective. Am J of Hospice Palliat Care 2001;18:251–5.

[23] Tilden VP, Tolle SW, Garland MJ, et al. Decisions about life-sustaining treatment: Impact of physicians' behaviors on the family. Arch Intern Med 1995;155(6): 633–8.

[24] Colen BD. Fight over life; Against family wishes, a Minnesota hospital may go to court in an effort to end measures keeping a woman alive by artificial means. *Newsday* (Nassau ed.), Jan 29, 1991. In Daar JF: A clash at the bedside: Patient autonomy v. a physician's professional conscience. *Hastings Law Journal* 1992–1993;44:1242.

[25] Cranford RE. Helga Wanglie's Ventilator. *Hastings Center Rep.*, July-Aug 1991, p. 23. In: Daar JF: A clash at the bedside: Patient autonomy v. a physician's professional conscience. *Hastings Law Journal* 1992–1993;44:1242.

[26] In re *Quinlan,* 355 A. 2d 647 (N.J. 1976).

[27] Edelstein L. *In Ancient Medicine: Selected Papers of Ludwig Edelstein.* Temkin O, Temkin CL (eds.): Baltimore, MD, Johns Hopkins Press, 1967, pp97–98. In The Ethics Committee of the Society of Critical Care of Medicine: Consensus statement of the Society of Critical Care Medicine's Ethics Committee regarding futile and other possibly inadvisable treatments. *Crit Care Med* 1997;25:887–991.

[28] Shevell MI. Reflections on futility. Semin Pediatr Neurol 2002;9:41–5.

[29] Lantos JD, Singer PA, Walker RM, et al. The illusion of futility in clinical practice. Am J Med 1989;87:81–4.

[30] Shannon TA, Walter JJ. Artificial nutrition, hydration: Assessing papal statement. Natl Cathol Report 2004;(April):16.

[31] Kelly SJG. Medico Moral Problems. St. Louis, Catholic Hospital Association, 1958, p.135. In The Ethics Committee of the Society of Critical Care of Medicine: Consensus statement of the Society of Critical Care Medicine's Ethics Committee regarding futile and other possibly inadvisable treatments. Crit Care Med 1997;25:887–991.

[32] President's Commission for the Study of Ethical Problems in Medicine and Biomedical and Behavioral Research Deciding to Forego Life-Sustaining Treatment. Washington D.C., US Government Printing Office, 1983, p. 219. In Shevell MI: Reflections on futility. Semin Pediatr Neurol 2002;9:41–5.

[33] *Cruzan v Director, Missouri Department of Health*, 497 US 261, 110 S Ct 2841 (1990).

[34] Federal Self-Determination Act 1990. 42 U.S.C. 1395 cc (a).

[35] *Superintendent of Belchertown v. Saikewicz* 370 N.E.2d 417 (Mass. 1977) In Daar JF: A clash at the

bedside: Patient autonomy v. a physician's professional conscience. *Hastings Law Journal* 1992–1993; 44:1261.

[36] *Payton v. Weaver*, 182 Cal. Rptr. 225, 229 (Cal. Ct. App. 1982). In Daar JF: A clash at the bedside: Patient autonomy v. a physician's professional conscience. *Hastings Law Journal* 1992–1993;44:1264.

[37] *Conservatorship of Morrison v. Abramovice*, 253 Cal. Rptr. 530 (Cal. Ct. App. 1988) In Daar JF: A clash at the bedside: Patient autonomy v. a physician's professional conscience. *Hastings Law Journal* 1992–1993;44:1267.

[38] *Brophy v. New England Sinai Hospital*, 497 N.E.2d 626 (Mass. 1986) In Daar JF: A clash at the bedside: Patient autonomy v. a physician's professional conscience. *Hastings Law Journal* 1992–1993;44:1268.

[39] VA. Code Ann. § 54.1–2990 (1994).

[40] MD. Code Ann., Health-Gen. §§ 5–601–618 (1994).

[41] Texas Health & Safety Code § 166.046 (2003). See also § 166.052 (2003).

[42] Cal Prob Code §4736 (West 2000). In Cantor MD, Braddock CH, Derse AR, et al.: Do-Not-Resuscitate orders and medical futility. *Arch Intern Med* 2003;163: 2689–94.

[43] California Probate Code § 4734–4735 (1999). Available: http://www.clrc.ca.gov/pub/publishers/1999-OfficialComments/99Cmts-B.rtf. [Accessed on March 20, 2005.]

[44] *Gilgunn v. Massachusetts General Hospital.* No 92–4820 (Mass. Sup. Ct. Civ. Action Suffolk Co. 22 Apr 1995).

[45] *Bryan v Rectors and Visitors of the University of Virginia*, 95 F3d 349 (4th Cir 1996).

[46] *Causey v. St. Francis Medical Center*, 710 So.2d 1072, 30,732 La. App. 2 Cir (1998).

[47] Peters PG. When physicians balk at futile care: Implications of the disability rights laws. Northwest Univ Law Rev 1997;91:827–30.

[48] Burt R. Resolving disputes between clinicians and family about "futility" of treatment. Semin Perinatol 2003;27:495–502.

[49] Daar JF: A clash at the bedside: Patient autonomy v. a physician's professional conscience. *Hastings Law Journal* 1992–1993;44:1241–89.

[50] *In re Baby K*, 16 F3d 590 (4th Cir. 1994).

[51] *In re Jobes*, 108 NJ 394, 529 A.2d 434 (1987).

[52] *Bartling v. Superior Court*, 209 Cal. Rptr. 220 (Cal.Ct. App 1984).

[53] Cantor NL. Can healthcare providers obtain judicial intervention against surrogates who demand 'medically inappropriate' life support for incompetent patients? Crit Care Med 1996;24(5):883–7.

[54] *In re Jane Doe*, 262 Ga. 389; 418 S.E. 2d 3; 1992.

[55] Kowalczyk L. Hospital, family spar over end-of-life care. Boston.com March 11, 2005. http://search.boston.com/index.jsp?queryStr=hospital%2C+family+spar+over+end-of-life+care&collection=month&title=c Accessed on March 16, 2005.]

[56] *In re Guardianship of Myers*, 610 N. E. 2d 663 (Ohio Misc. 1993).

[57] Bopp J, Coleson RE. Child abuse by whom?—Parental rights and judicial competency determinations: The Baby K and Baby Terry Cases. Ohio NU L Rev 1994; 821:825–7.

[58] Haidar S, Cerminara K. *Key events in the case of Theresa Marie Schiavo*. Available: http://www.miami.edu/ethics2/schiavo/timeline.htm. [Accessed on April 5, 2005.]

[59] Field MJ, Behrman R (eds). *Institute of Medicine, When Children Die: Improving Palliative and End-of-Life Care for Children and Their Families*. Washington, DC, National Academy Press, 2002, p. 293. In Burt R: Resolving disputes between clinicians and family about "futility" of treatment. Semin Perinatol 2003;27:495–502.

[60] Abbott KH, Sago JG, Breen CM, et al. Families looking back: One year after discussion of withdrawal or withholding of life-sustaining support. Crit Care Med 2001;29:197–201.

[61] Kowalczyk L. Hospital, family agree to withdraw life support. Boston.com March 12, 2005. Available: http://search.boston.com/index.jsp?queryStr=hospital%2C+family+spar+over+end-of-life+care&collection=month&title=c [Accessed on March 16, 2005.]

[62] Schneiderman LJ, Gilmer T, Teetzel HD, et al. Effect of ethics consultations on nonbeneficial life-sustaining treatments in the intensive care setting: A randomized controlled trial. JAMA 2003;290:1166–72.

[63] Council on Ethical and Judicial Affairs. American Medical Association: Medical Futility in End-of-Life Care: Report of the Council on Ethical and Judicial Affairs. JAMA 1999;281(10):937–41.

[64] Casarett D, Siegler M. Unilateral do-not-attempt-resuscitation orders and ethics consultation: a case series. Crit Care Med 1999;27(6):1116–20.

[65] Orentlicher D. Futility as a way to make "tragic choices." In: Orentlicher D, editor. Matters of life and death: Making moral theory work in medical ethics and the law. Princeton (NJ): Princeton University Press; 2001. p. 164.

[66] Weijer C, Singer PA, Dickens BM, et al. Bioethics for clinicians: Dealing with demands for inappropriate treatment. CMAJ 1998;159:817–22.

[67] Bone RC, Rackow EC, Weg JG, et al. Ethical and moral guidelines for the initiation, continuation, and withdrawal of intensive care. Chest 1990;97:949–58.

[68] American Academy of Neurology (AAN). Guidelines on the vegetative state: Commentary on the AAN statement and position of the AAN on certain aspects of the care and management of the persistent vegetative state. Neurology 1989;39:123–6.

[69] American Thoracic Society. Withholding and Withdrawing life-sustaining therapy. Am Rev Respir Dis 1991;144:726–31.

[70] Daar JF. Medical futility and implications for physician autonomy. Am J Law Med 1995;21:221–40.

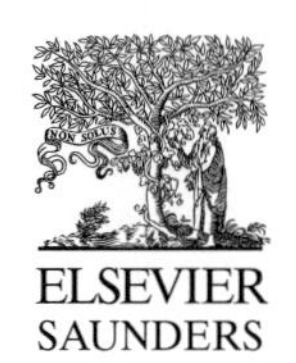
ELSEVIER
SAUNDERS

Thorac Surg Clin 15 (2005) 493 – 501

THORACIC
SURGERY
CLINICS

Ethical Issues in Patient Safety

Lucian L. Leape, MD

Harvard School of Public Health, Department of Health Policy and Management, 677 Huntington Avenue, Boston, MA 02215, USA

In 1999, the Institute of Medicine (IOM) published a landmark report, "To Err is Human," that shocked America with the revelation that as many as 98,000 people die annually as the result of medical errors [1]. Although some have questioned the validity of the mortality estimate [2,3], few still question the seriousness of the problem of medical errors and injuries or the need to do something about it [4–6].

In addition to the shocking numbers, the IOM report advanced the thesis, long accepted by students of error, that most mistakes that are made by individuals are caused by systems failures, not by individual carelessness or incompetence. This new look calls for a radical realignment of efforts to prevent injuries: away from an exclusive focus on the individual to an examination of the systems in health care. The IOM called for a nonpunitive approach to errors and a massive national effort to redesign health care systems to make them safer.

Adverse events, defined as injuries caused by medical treatment as contrasted with complications of disease, are distressingly common in hospitalized patients. Multiple population-based studies have shown rates varying from 3% to 13% of admissions [7–10]. Many of these are unavoidable and are well-known complications of treatment that we are unable to prevent at the current level of scientific knowledge. These include such complications as a first-time allergic reaction to a new drug, wound infections following contaminated surgery, some postoperative thromboembolic episodes, arrhythmias, and so forth. Elimination of these complications comes, as it has come with other complications in former times, through advances in the science and practice of medicine and surgery.

A greater proportion of adverse events, probably two thirds of the total, are avoidable [8–12]. These are injuries that result from substandard performance; equipment failures; and, by far the most common (probably 90%–95% of the total), mistakes made by well-trained, highly skilled, conscientious practitioners. It is these that the new look, or systems theory, addresses.

The systems approach to preventing medical errors

Systems theory holds that individuals are set up to make mistakes by faulty design of the processes we work in; conditions under which we work (including schedules, work loads, and hours); management and leadership styles; physical surroundings; equipment design and maintenance; and other factors [13]. There are two corollaries to this theory: first, that one can prevent mistakes by redesigning systems, and second, that it makes no sense to punish the individual who makes a mistake. Punishing the individual does not keep another person from making the same mistake later; only changing the system does that [12].

Evidence has now accumulated in health care to support both of these assertions: systems changes are effective in reducing errors, and creation of a nonpunitive environment greatly expands reporting of errors and leads to expanded efforts to identify underlying systems causes and correct them. A few examples of systems changes:

- Some years ago occasional patients died during anesthesia as a result of erroneous connection of

E-mail address: leape@hsph.harvard.edu

1547-4127/05/$ – see front matter
doi:10.1016/j.thorsurg.2005.06.007

the nitrous oxide tank to the oxygen port of the anesthesia machine. Redesigning the connectors to make this impossible eliminated the error, and deaths [14].

- Until recently, each year 8 to 15 patients (the exact number will never be known) died because of accidental intravenous injection of concentrated potassium chloride. Concentrated potassium chloride was widely available "on the shelf" in nursing units for ease of addition to intravenous infusions. Mix-ups were exceedingly rare, but did happen, with devastating effect. Removing concentrated potassium chloride from the units, requiring potassium chloride to be added by the pharmacy (or provided in premixed intravenous bags) has virtually eliminated this tragedy [15].
- Handwritten orders are prone to misinterpretation: QD read as QID, 1.0 read as 10, and so forth. Enforcement of strict rules on use of abbreviations, prohibition of "trailing zeroes," and so forth can reduce these errors. Computerizing the ordering process is even more effective, and has been shown to reduce serious medication errors by 80% [16]. Both are systems changes that are far more likely to prevent errors than exhorting doctors and nurses to be more careful.

Progress in changing systems

Five years after the IOM report and 10 years after the true beginning of the patient safety movement in health care following a series of highly publicized medical mistakes in 1995 and the first demonstrations of the application of systems theory in health care [17] a nationwide effort is well under way to make health care safer by redesigning practically all of our systems [18]. The National Quality Forum has identified 30 safe practices, feasible changes in procedures that have been demonstrated to reduce errors (Box 1) [19], and the Joint Commission for the Accreditation of Healthcare Organizations (JCAHO) has begun to require hospitals to implement these and other safe practices [20,21].

The Accreditation Council for Graduate Medical Education has implemented a restriction of resident duty hours to 80 hours per week to reduce hazard caused by fatigue and sleeplessness. Although this change has created a new set of problems related to coverage and education, the need for it is clear [22]. Together with the American Board of Medical Specialties, the Accreditation Council for Graduate Medical Education has begun the development of the definitions of competencies, including in safety, and measures to be used for assessing residents and diplomates in practice to ensure safe and competent practice.

Taking the lead from aviation, many institutions and systems (including Kaiser Permanente and the Veterans Health Administration) have instituted team training programs [23,24]. Payers have entered the mix, linking reimbursement to implementation of safe practices, such as requiring intensive care units to have a full-time intensivist, limiting high-risk surgery to institutions with sufficient volume of cases, and implementation of computerized ordering systems [25].

The implications of the systems approach are profound and far-reaching. Some of the most important are as follows:

1. When mishaps occur, do not blame the individual; look for the underlying causes, known as "contributing factors" or root causes, which are always multiple.
2. Systems need to be redesigned using human factors principles that make it easy for the individual to perform a task correctly and difficult to do it wrong. Almost all systems and processes in health care benefit from redesign.
3. Hospitals have a clear obligation to take all practical steps that are known to improve safety; specifically, they should promptly implement known safe practices, as defined by the JCAHO and the National Quality Forum.
4. Regulators and accreditors have a fiduciary responsibility to the public to hold hospitals accountable to make these changes to improve safety.
5. Safety is a property of systems and relationships. No system can be safe unless personnel work well together and every individual in an organization believes they are personally responsible for safety: responsible to implement safe practices, to follow safe practices, and to identify hazards.

Problems with the systems approach

Not surprisingly, there has been "push back" by physicians and others concerning this new look. Some have been concerned that shifting the focus to systems will lead to irresponsible behavior ("Don't blame me, the system made me do it!"). This is a

Box 1. National Quality Forum – endorsed set of safe practices

1. Create a healthcare culture of safety.
2. For designated high-risk, elective surgical procedures or other specified care, patients should be clearly informed of the likely reduced risk of an adverse outcome at treatment facilities that have demonstrated superior outcomes and should be referred to such facilities in accordance with the patient's stated preference.
3. Specify an explicit protocol to be used to ensure an adequate level of nursing based on the institution's usual patient mix and the experience and training of its nursing staff.
4. All patients in general intensive care units (both adult and pediatric) should be managed by physicians having specific training and certification in critical care medicine (''critical care certified'').
5. Pharmacists should actively participate in the medication-use process, including, at a minimum, being available for consultation with prescribers on medication ordering, interpretation and review of medication orders, preparation of medications, dispensing of medications, and administration and monitoring of medications.
6. Verbal orders should be recorded whenever possible and immediately read back to the prescriber -i.e., a healthcare provider receiving a verbal order should read or repeat back the information that the prescriber conveys in order to verify the accuracy of what was heard.
7. Use only standardized abbreviations and dose designations.
8. Patient care summaries or other similar records should not be prepared from memory.
9. Ensure that care information, especially changes in orders and new diagnostic information, is transmitted in a timely and clearly understandable form to all of the patient's current healthcare providers who need that information to provide care.
10. Ask each patient or legal surrogate to recount what he or she has been told during the informed consent discussion.
11. Ensure that written documentation of the patient's preference for life-sustaining treatments is prominently displayed in his or her chart.
12. Implement a computerized prescriber order entry system.
13. Implement a standardized protocol to prevent the mislabeling of radiographs.
14. Implement standardized protocols to prevent the occurrence of wrong-site procedures or wrong-patient procedures.
15. Evaluate each patient undergoing elective surgery for risk of an acute ischemic cardiac event during surgery, and provide prophylactic treatment of high-risk patients with beta blockers.
16. Evaluate each patient upon admission, and regularly thereafter, for the risk *of* developing pressure ulcers. This evaluation should be repeated at regular intervals during care. Clinically appropriate preventive methods should be implemented consequent to the evaluation.
17. Evaluate each patient upon admission, and regularly thereafter, for the risk of developing deep vein thrombosis (DVT)/venous thromboembolism (VTE). Utilize clinically appropriate methods to prevent DVT/VTE.
18. Utilize dedicated anti-thrombotic (anti-coagulation) services that facilitate coordinated care management.
19. Upon admission, and regularly thereafter, evaluate each patient for the risk of aspiration.
20. Adhere to effective methods of preventing central venous catheter-associated blood stream infections.
21. Evaluate each pre-operative patient in light of his or her planned surgical procedure for the risk of surgical site infection, and implement appropriate antibiotic prophylaxis and other preventive measures based on that evaluation.

22. Utilize validated protocols to evaluate patients who are at risk for contrast media-induced renal failure, and utilize a clinically appropriate method for reducing risk of renal injury based on the patient's kidney function evaluation.
23. Evaluate each patient upon admission, and regularly thereafter, for risk of malnutrition. Employ clinically appropriate strategies to prevent malnutrition.
24. Whenever a pneumatic tourniquet is used, evaluate the patient for the risk of an ischemic and/or thrombotic complication, and utilize appropriate prophylactic measures.
25. Decontaminate hands with either a hygienic hand rub or by washing with a disinfectant soap prior to and after direct contact with the patient or objects immediately around the patient.
26. Vaccinate healthcare workers against influenza to protect both them and patients from influenza.
27. Keep workspaces where medications are prepared clean, orderly, well lit, and free of clutter, distraction, and noise.
28. Standardize the methods for labeling, packaging, and storing medications.
29. Identify all ''high alert'' drugs (e.g., intravenous adrenergic agonists and antagonists, chemotherapy agents, anticoagulants and anti-thrombotics, concentrated parenteral electrolytes, general anesthetics, neuromuscular blockers, insulin and oral hypoglycemics, narcotics and opiates).
30. Dispense medications in unit-dose or, when appropriate, unit-of-use form, whenever possible.

See full report for applicable care settings for each practice, detailed specifications, and additional background and reference material.

Safe Practices for Better Healthcare: A Consensus Report. © 2003 National Quality Forum, www.qualityforum.org, Washington, DC; with permission.

misunderstanding of the theory. When a major error occurs, the individual at the "sharp end" (the one who made the mistake) has a much higher responsibility than just to take his or her punishment. That person has a responsibility both to report the event and to participate in an investigation to understand the underlying systems failures. He or she has unique knowledge of the event that is essential to its understanding. A nonpunitive environment empowers individuals to come forth and take this responsibility rather than to hide and hope it will not be uncovered.

Accountability

Many confuse "nonpunitive" with "blame-free." Systems theory holds that individuals should not be punished for errors. But a safe system also requires accountability; misconduct cannot be tolerated. The important point is to recognize that errors are not misconduct. Misconduct is deliberate violation of rules and procedures, such as refusal to follow procedures for correct site identification, refusal to get a radiograph when a sponge count is incorrect, or other established standards of performance. In a culture of safety, this type of behavior is not tolerated [26,27]. Abusive behavior is also considered misconduct because of its corrosive effect on the performance of others.

Malpractice

The threat of malpractice litigation is another barrier to acceptance and implementation of systems theory. Many physicians are reluctant to report or talk about their mistakes because of fear that it increases the likelihood of their being sued for malpractice. Although in the present litigious climate this is understandable, it is based on a myth. Not only is internal discussion of errors protected from discovery, there is no evidence that admission of a mistake to the patient increases the likelihood of being sued. In fact, just the contrary seems to be so.

Regulatory lag

The regulatory apparatus often lags behind advances in thinking about managing mistakes, and can be a substantial barrier to an open and systems-based approach to medical errors. Although the JCAHO has been forward-thinking, many state health departments are less so. Most state medical boards function in a reactive mode, seeing their role as punishing errant doctors rather than becoming involved in influencing hospitals to create environments where substandard performance is less likely to occur.

For all these reasons, progress in improving patient safety has been halting and slow. The pace of change is accelerating, however, as most of these barriers turn out to be in fact far less significant than many had presumed.

Ethical concerns

Ethical concerns related to patient safety can be classified into four main categories:

1. The imperative to implement and follow safe practices
2. Responding to adverse events
3. Responding to the injured patient
4. Taking responsibility for problem doctors

The imperative to implement and follow safe practices

An important objective of a system seeking to be safe is to implement practices and procedures that are known to minimize the likelihood of complications, such as infection or mistaken identity, and to ensure that all personnel follow them: to "do the right thing." As hospitals have become more committed to improving patient safety, both implementation and enforcement of safe practices has turned out to be a huge challenge.

The ethical issue around safe practice is straightforward: we have a moral obligation to our patients to do everything reasonably possible to make care safe: first, do no harm. How can we ethically do otherwise? Our patients trust us to ensure safe care to the extent we are able. Clearly, we should do everything within our power and resources to honor that trust. Curiously, this aspect of ethical behavior is rarely discussed.

The practical issues can be daunting. Health care is incredibly complex; we have much to learn about how to redesign our systems to make them safe. There is a lot, however, that we do know. There are many specific practices that are known to make a difference in safety. The National Quality Forum list of 30 is based on evidence of effectiveness and real world experience in implementation (see Box 1) [19]. Yet, as far as the author has been able to ascertain, no hospital has implemented them all, and most hospitals have implemented only a few, usually reluctantly, and only under fear of JCAHO sanction.

There are always many reasons for sluggishness in changing practices, including almost always limited resources. Yet, hospitals that are serious about safety find ways to get them done. It is a matter of priorities: hospitals usually find resources to purchase a new MRI machine, or establish a catheterization laboratory.

On the implementation side, a great deal of effort and discussion in quality improvement circles revolves around theories of how to persuade physicians to change behavior (ie, implement a new process or protocol, such as by providing data, enlisting champions, starting on a small scale, and so forth). From an ethical standpoint, the question is much simpler: how can an individual physician justify placing his or her own judgment or preference over a reasoned institutional decision to implement a new safe practice that national experts have recommended based on careful review of the evidence?

An equally sticky ethical issue is compliance, following safe practices. How can a physician justify not observing a safe practice, knowing that failure to do so exposes some patients to increased risk of injury? The answers are not simple. Consider hand hygiene (eg, disinfecting one's hands before and after touching a patient). The evidence for effectiveness of this practice in reducing nosocomial infections, particularly those caused by resistant organisms, is powerful [28]. Yet, compliance by physicians is typically less than 50%.

There are many reasons for the failure of hand hygiene practice. The relationship between failure and infection is not one-to-one; most times the uncleansed doctor does not infect the patient; the doctor is in a hurry; he or she just disinfected after the previous patient; he or she "will not touch the patient" (just the record, or the table, or coat, tie, stethoscope, pen, handkerchief); and so forth. The practical arguments are many: justifications; rationalizations; even (increasingly indefensible) doubts about effectiveness.

The ethical argument is simple: if the evidence is clear, and it is, then the only morally defensible action is 100% compliance. The question becomes how to do it, not whether. It is worth noting that this argument was settled a century ago, on the basis of much less evidence, with regard to hand disinfection before performing surgery.

Responding to adverse events

How an organization, and the individuals in it, responds to a serious adverse event is a measure of its commitment to safety. Defensive, insecure hospitals regard bad news as threats to their reputation and seek to conceal or minimize them. Open, responsible, "learning" organizations that are committed to safety look on a serious adverse event as a symptom of a failed system [29]. It is a wake up call, an opportunity for improvement. They want to understand what happened and do what it takes to make sure it does not happen again.

There are several levels of ethical responsibility. The first level is regarding the patient. The injured patient has a right to know what happened. As the party responsible for the injury, the institution has an obligation to find out where things broke down and provide an explanation. The second level is to future patients: what can be learned so that changes can be made to keep a similar event from happening to other patients in this hospital in the future. The third level is to patients everywhere: lessons learned should be disseminated broadly (as by a state or JCAHO sentinel events reporting system) to other hospitals to enable them to make changes to prevent similar mishaps on future patients.

None of this can happen unless events are reported when they occur. The first ethical obligation for the individual physician is to report mishaps: adverse events caused by errors or other systems failures, and serious near miss errors that represent potential hazards to future patients. An open, non-punitive, well-used reporting system is a cornerstone of an ethical response to adverse events. Physicians also have an obligation to participate in the investigation to understand what systems failed and why. Finally, they have an obligation to inform the patient of the findings and explain what is being done to prevent recurrence. All of these steps are essential parts of a meaningful safety system. All have ethical implications.

The hospital's ethical obligation is, when possible, to make those necessary systems changes and provide the information to higher authorities for dissemination. These higher authorities (state health departments and the JCAHO) in turn have an ethical obligation to disseminate lessons learned broadly, so all hospitals benefit from them. The ethical obligations of regulators are not a subject that is often discussed. Perhaps it should be.

Responding to the injured patient

A revered student of medical mishaps, British psychologist Charles Vincent, has observed that medical injury differs from other types of trauma in two ways. First, patients are unintentionally harmed by the people in whom they have placed trust. Second, they usually continue to be cared for by the same clinicians who were involved in the injury itself, which can cause conflicting feelings about their caregivers [30].

When they are injured by physicians' mistakes, patients may feel hurt, betrayed, devalued, humiliated, and afraid. Anxiety, depression, anger, frustration, and feelings of isolation are not uncommon reactions [30,31]. A preventable adverse event is a major threat to a patient's trust.

What do patients want? Experience from mediation of cases where patients have filed malpractice claims shows patients consistently have three common objectives: (1) to find out what happened, (2) to hear the doctor say he or she is sorry, and (3) to be assured that something has been done to prevent the same thing from happening to someone else. These findings are consistent with results of patient surveys. Most patients wish to be informed of adverse events when they happen. In a survey conducted among 149 patients from a United States academic internal medicine outpatient clinic [32], patients were asked to respond to medical error scenarios. Ninety-eight percent wanted some acknowledgment of errors, even if they were minor, and most indicated they were significantly more likely to consider litigation if the physician did not disclose the error.

The ethical imperative is clear: the Golden Rule applies. Patients are entitled to a full and truthful explanation of what happened. There is no moral justification for withholding information or misrepresenting the facts. It is imperative, however, that only the facts that are known be communicated. Early after a mishap, reasons for it may be unclear, so the explanation should be confined to explaining what happened, not why. Further explanation should be provided later after the investigation is completed.

In most cases, the patient's physician is responsible for providing the explanations, even if the injury was caused by actions of another. When the injury results from a clear-cut mistake by the physician, he or she should take responsibility for it and apologize.

By taking responsibility and apologizing, the physician acknowledges the patient's feelings of anger and loss of trust, shows an understanding of their impact, and begins to make amends. Apology helps to restore the patient's dignity and begins the healing process [33]. Apologizing also helps the physician deal with his or her own emotional trauma, which can be substantial.

In follow-up conversations, it is important to inform the patient and family of what the investigation reveals and what the plans are for changes to prevent recurrence. Caregivers often underestimate the extent to which injured patients have a strong interest in seeing to it that what happened to them does not happen to someone else. Knowing that changes were made and that some good came of their experience helps the patient and family cope with their pain or loss. It gives a positive meaning to their experience to know that their suffering is not in vain.

What about the malpractice risk of full disclosure and apologizing? From an ethical standpoint, whether or not disclosure leads to an increased risk of being sued is irrelevant. After all, the first tenant of professionalism is to put the interests of your patient above your own. Although this is the ideal, achieving it can be difficult. For years, physicians have been counseled by hospital lawyers not to admit that anything went wrong, not to take responsibility, and above all never to apologize.

It has seemed logical to assume that doing so increases the likelihood that the patient will sue. The facts seem to be just the reverse. Not only is there no evidence that being honest with patients or apologizing increases the risk of being sued, there is abundant anecdotal evidence that physicians' failure to be honest, take responsibility, and show remorse are major reasons why patients file suits. Recently, quantitative evidence has seemed to support openness in disclosure: in the Veterans' Health Administration [34,35], at the University of Michigan [36], and among COPIC insured in Colorado. In all of these early experiences, open, honest, full disclosure, sometimes coupled with small payments, has led to fewer suits and lower overall payments. It seems that full disclosure is not only the right thing to do, it is the smart thing to do. From an ethical standpoint, however, full disclosure and apology is required even if it were to increase the rate and costs of litigation.

Taking responsibility for problem doctors

The IOM may proclaim that errors are caused by bad systems, not bad people, but the public remains unconvinced. Repeated surveys show that most people think the medical injury problem is caused by incompetent doctors, and that if those doctors were removed care would be safe.

Although the public may be wrong (certainly most students of error prevention believe they are) the fact is that there are some doctors whose performance is unacceptable, and an even larger group who have problems from time to time that may lead to unsafe practice. Within the profession these issues are not dealt with very well, often not at all.

What are the facts? Leaving aside the very rare psychopathic or sociopathic personality disorders that occasionally get headlines, many physicians are at risk of impaired performance. Physician performance can be dangerously substandard at one time or another during one's career as a result of any of a number of factors: drug or alcohol abuse (estimated to afflict 5% and 10%, respectively) [37]; mental illness (15% lifetime risk) [38]; physical illness (approximately 5%–10% lifetime risk); reduced competency (no valid measures available, but probably 5%–10%); and abusive or disruptive behavior (5% of physicians) [39,40]. Even allowing for overlap of categories, it seems that 30% to 40% of physicians may suffer from a condition that, at some time during their practice, significantly impairs performance and poses a threat to patient safety. Most receive little help.

Failure to ensure competent and safe practice of all of our colleagues is an ethical lapse of major proportions for our profession. The public entrusts us to ensure quality. No one else can do it. Our professional credo pledges us to do it. We claim the right to freedom from external oversight based on a commitment to self-regulation. Yet we do not do it. Why?

The reasons are complex. One is that we tend to think reactively: how to respond when doctors go bad, not how to prevent it. Understandably, we are loathe to act until it is absolutely necessary. Second, it seems to be an "all or nothing" proposition: either we remove privileges (and means of earning a livelihood) or we do nothing. We see few intermediate alternatives. Third, we all live in glass houses; no one is perfect, who am I to judge, and so forth. Finally, and most important, we do not have a good system for identifying and helping physicians who need help. In the absence of a system for objectively identifying physicians in trouble, evaluations are often based on ad hoc, anecdotal, subjective judgments that are understandably open to challenge. To discharge our ethical responsibility to protect the public and help our colleagues, we need better systems.

Developing such systems is not easy, but it must be done. Many tools are already available for assessing competency, disruptive behavior, and identifying physicians with mental disorders or substance abuse. A relatively simple but powerful overall measure is the use of "360" evaluations, as has been pioneered by the Physician Achievement Review program in Alberta, Canada [41]. Hospital staffs (and practices) need to implement routine, regular (annual) review of all physicians; identify those needing help; and provide counseling, remedial training, or other assistance. Rarely, individuals are refractory to treatment, in which case their practice must be promptly curtailed. Legally robust mechanisms must be established to achieve these objectives.

The practical aspects of developing effective and fair methods for routine assessment of physician performance are complex, but not insurmountable. As with many of the other issues in patient safety, the ethical imperative is much simpler: we owe it to the public and all of our patients to take the steps necessary to ensure that all physicians are safe and competent.

Summary

Making progress in patient safety poses many challenges, practical and theoretical, to the way physicians practice medicine. The ethical challenges are among the most profound. They include the ethical imperative to do all things practical to prevent errors and injury to patients, the need to respond appropriately when things go wrong to find new methods to prevent recurrence, the requirement for honesty and openness in dealing with our patients when things go wrong, and taking responsibility for ensuring that all of our colleagues are safe and competent. This is an immense challenge. It is not easy to "first, do no harm." But only we as a profession can meet this challenge. No one else can do it; we must.

References

[1] Kohn KT, Corrigan JM, Donaldson MS, editors. To err is human: building a safer health system. Washington: National Academy Press; 1999.

[2] McDonald CJ, Weiner M, Hui SL. Deaths due to medical errors are exaggerated in Institute of Medicine report. JAMA 2000;284:93–4.

[3] Leape LL. Institute of Medicine medical error figures are not exaggerated. JAMA 2000;284:95–7.

[4] Starfield B. Is US health really the best in the world? JAMA 2000;284:483–5.

[5] Healey MA, Shackford SR, Osler TM, et al. Complications in surgical patients. Arch Surg 2002;137: 611–8.

[6] Zhan C, Miller M. Excess length of stay, charges, and mortality attributable to medical injuries during hospitalization. JAMA 2003;290:1868–74.

[7] Brennan TA, Leape LL, Laird N, et al. Incidence of adverse events and negligence in hospitalized patients: results from the Harvard medical practice study I. N Engl J Med 1991;324:370–6.

[8] Thomas EJ, Studdert DM, Burstin HR, et al. Incidence and types of adverse events and negligent care in Utah and Colorado. Med Care 2000;38:261–71.

[9] Wilson R, Runciman W, Gibberd R, et al. The quality in Australian health care study. Med J Aust 1995;163: 458–71.

[10] Vincent C, Neale G, Woloshynowych M. Adverse events in British hospitals: preliminary retrospective record review. BMJ 2001;322:517–9.

[11] Leape LL, Lawthers AG, Brennan TA, et al. Preventing medical injury. Quality Review Bulletin 1993;19: 144–9.

[12] Leape LL. Error in medicine. JAMA 1994;272: 1851–7.

[13] Reason J. Human error. Cambridge: Cambridge University Press; 1990.

[14] Pierce E. The 34th Rovenstine Lecture. 40 years behind the mask: safety revisited. Anesthesiology 1996; 84:965–75.

[15] JCAHO. Sentinel event trends: potassium chloride. Available at: http://www.jcaho.org/accredited+organizations/ambulatory+care/sentinel+events/set+potassium.htm. Accessed April 2, 2005.

[16] Bates DW, Teich JM, Lee J, et al. The impact of computerized physician order entry on medication error prevention. J Am Med Inform Assoc 1999;6: 313–21.

[17] Leape LL, Bates DW, Cullen DJ, et al. Systems analysis of adverse drug events. JAMA 1995;274:35–43.

[18] Leape LL, Berwick DM. Five years after "To Err Is Human" what have we learned? JAMA 2005;293: 2384–90.

[19] National Quality Forum. Safe practices for better health care: a consensus report. Report No. NQFCR-05–03. Washington (DC): National Quality Forum; 2003.

[20] JCAHO. New safety and error reduction standards for hospitals. Joint Comm Perspectives 2001;21:1–3.

[21] JCAHO. Joint Commission announces national patient safety goals. Available at: http://www.jcaho.org/news+room/latest+from+jcaho/npsg.htmv. Accessed December 3, 2002.

[22] Landrigan C, Rothchild J, Cronin J, et al. Effect of reducing interns' work hours on serious medical errors in intensive care units. N Engl J Med 2004;351: 1838–48.

[23] Helmreich D, Musson D. Surgery as team endeavor. Can J Anesth 2000;47:391–2.

[24] Bagian JP, Lee C, Gosbee J, et al. Developing and deploying a patient safety program in a large health care delivery system: you can't fix what you don't know about. Jt Comm J Qual Improv 2001;27:522–32.
[25] Milstein A, Galvin RS, Delbanco SF, et al. Improving the safety of health care: the Leapfrog Initiative. Eff Clin Pract 2000;3:313–6.
[26] Marx D. How building a "just culture" helps an organization learn from errors. OR Manager 2003;19(5):1, 14–5, 20.
[27] Reason JT. Managing the risks of organizational accidents. Brookfield (VT): Ashgate; 1997.
[28] Gerberding JL. Hospital-onset infections: a patient safety issue. Ann Intern Med 2002;137:665–70.
[29] Senge P. The fifth discipline: the art and practice of the learning organization. New York: Doubleday; 1990.
[30] Vincent C. Understanding and responding to adverse events. N Engl J Med 2003;348:1051–6.
[31] Vincent C, Young M, Phillips A. Why do people sue doctors? A study of patients and relatives taking legal action. Lancet 1994;343:1609–14.
[32] Witman AB, Park DM, Hardin SB. How do patients want physicians to handle mistakes? A survey of internal medicine patients in an academic setting. Arch Intern Med 1996;156:2565–9.
[33] Lazare A. On apology. New York: Oxford University Press; 2004.
[34] Kraman SS, Hamm G. Risk management: extreme honesty may be the best policy. Ann Intern Med 1999;131:963–7.
[35] Kachalia A, Shojania KG, Hofer TP, et al. Does full disclosure of medical errors affect malpractice liability? Jt Comm J Qual Saf 2003;29:503–11.
[36] Hall S. U-M docs say sorry, avert suits. Detroit News May 12, 2004.
[37] Lutsky I, Hopwood N, Abram SE, et al. The use of psychoactive substances in three medical specialties: anesthesia, medicine and surgery. Can J Anaesth 1994;41:561–7.
[38] Kessler RC, Berglund P, Demler O, et al. The epidemiology of major depressive disorder: results from the National Comorbidity Survey Replication (NCS-R). JAMA 2003;289:3095–105.
[39] Rosenstein A, O'Daniel M. Disruptive behavior and clinical outcomes: perceptions of nurses and physicians. Am J Nursing 2005;105:54–64.
[40] Linney BJ. Confronting the disruptive physician. Physician Exec 1997;23:55–8.
[41] College of Physicians and Surgeons of Alberta. Physician achievement review. 2004. Available at: www.par-program.org. Accessed October 23, 2004.

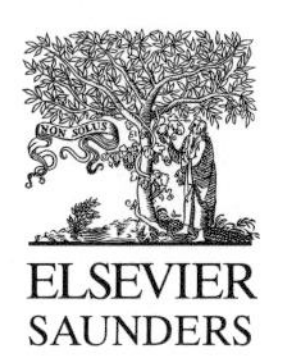
ELSEVIER
SAUNDERS

Thorac Surg Clin 15 (2005) 503 – 512

THORACIC
SURGERY
CLINICS

Solving the Problem of the Uninsured

John C. Goodman, PhD

National Center for Policy Analysis, 12770 Coit Road, Suite 800, Dallas, TX 75251–1339, USA

The fact that millions of Americans do not have health insurance is said to be a major problem, if not the major problem, of the United States health care system. Estimates of the number who are uninsured vary widely. There are also widely different indicators of how much difference uninsurance makes. Proposed solutions range from single-payer national health insurance to individual or employer mandates to tax subsidies for the purchase of private health insurance. Even the proponents admit these proposals require large taxpayer burdens and new federal bureaucracies.

Fortunately, there is a way to deal with this problem that does not require new taxes or cumbersome (and probably unenforceable) mandates. Nor does the solution require the knowledge of how many uninsured there are at any one time or what difference uninsurance makes. The solution involves integrating the current system of tax subsidies (which encourage people to obtain private insurance) with the system of spending subsidies (which encourage people not to be insured). The purpose of the integration is to ensure that government policies are not encouraging people to be uninsured, and causing the very problem that needs to be solved.

All physicians are familiar with the do-no-harm principle in medical ethics. It is time to apply that same principle to public policy.

Nature of the problem

The latest Census Bureau report estimates that 45 million Americans are uninsured at any one time [1]. Yet, estimates using the Census Bureau's Survey of Income and Program Participation suggest that the actual number of uninsured could be half as large. For instance, a Congressional Budget Office study of the Census Bureau's Survey of Income and Program Participation estimated the actual number of uninsured may be as low as 21 million [2]. Another report finds that, even using Census Bureau methods, the 45 million number is about 25% too high, or off by 9 million people [3].

Regardless of the actual number, what is more important is how long people are uninsured. Being uninsured is like being unemployed. Most people probably experience the condition over the course of a lifetime, but in most cases it is temporary. Very few people are uninsured for a long period of time. For instance, 75% of uninsured spells are over within 12 months. Less than 10% last longer than 2 years [4].

There are dozens of studies that claim to find significant health differences between those who are insured and those who are uninsured. For instance, Marquis and Long [5,6] find that uninsured adults have about 60% as many physician visits and 70% as many inpatient hospital days as they would if they were covered by insurance. Yet, there are reasons to doubt these results. Consider the fact that there are between 10 and 14 million people who are theoretically eligible for Medicaid and SCHIP (for low-income families who do not qualify for Medicaid) but do not bother to sign up. This is almost one in every four uninsured persons in the country. Estimates of eligibility for public health care programs vary. The

The original title was modified to this version by the request of the Guest Editor, Dr. Sade.

E-mail address: jcgoodman@ncpa.org

1547-4127/05/$ – see front matter
doi:10.1016/j.thorsurg.2005.06.010

lower estimates are that around 10 million Americans are eligible but unenrolled, whereas the upper range of estimates is closer to 14 million. One study found that just over half (51.4%) of eligible, nonelderly adults were enrolled in Medicaid in 1997. Of the remaining adults who were Medicaid eligible, 21.6% had private coverage, whereas 27% were uninsured. Another study found that about 7 million uninsured children eligible for either SCHIP or Medicaid are not enrolled [7]. Of those children eligible for Medicaid or SCHIP, one third is eligible for SCHIP, whereas two thirds are eligible for Medicaid. Eight percent of uninsured, low-income children are illegal aliens and, as such, not eligible for either Medicaid or SCHIP [8,9]. Furthermore, in most places people are able to enroll in Medicaid up to 3 months after they receive medical treatment. Because these people can enroll at the drop of a hat, even after they have incurred medical expenses, are they not de facto insured even without the necessity of formal enrollment?

To see what this means on the local level, consider Parkland Hospital in Dallas, a primary source of care for the indigent and those covered by Medicaid. Uninsured patients and Medicaid patients pass through the same emergency room door; they see the same doctors; they receive the same treatments; and if required, they are admitted to hospital rooms on the same floors [10].

The only people who seem to care very much about who is insured or uninsured at Parkland are the hospital staff (presumably because that affects how they get paid). For that reason, full-time employees work their way through the emergency room waiting area to enroll all eligible patients in Medicaid (most of the time they fail). With the same goal in mind, employees also go room to room to visit those who are admitted (where their success rate is much higher).

At Children's Medical Center, next door to Parkland, a similar exercise takes place. Children on Medicaid, children on SCHIP, and uninsured children all come through the same emergency room door. Again, they all see the same doctors and receive the same treatments. Again, it is only the hospital that seems to care whether anybody is insured and by whom [10].

If a $100 bill were dropped on the emergency room floor at Parkland, it probably would not remain there for 60 seconds; but an application to enroll in Medicaid dropped on the same floor might remain there for hours. In the view of some commentators, the enrollment forms are a ticket to health insurance worth thousands of dollars and substantially more health care. But people do not act as thought they believe that is the case. To the contrary, they act as though the marginal value of enrollment is virtually zero.

For the millions of people who opt not to enroll in free government-provided health insurance, uninsurance is the result of voluntary choice. A lot of other people are also voluntarily uninsured. For example, about 9 million people (more than one in five of the uninsured) are eligible for employer insurance and decline to enroll even though the employee share of the premium is usually nominal [11].

It can be inferred that many other people are voluntarily uninsured, because they apparently have enough income to purchase insurance if they choose. Although it is common to think of the uninsured as having low incomes, many families who lack insurance are solidly middle class (Fig. 1). The largest increase in the number of uninsured in recent years has occurred among higher-income families. About one in three uninsured persons (14.8 million people) lives in a family with an income of $50,000 or higher and about half of those have incomes in excess of $75,000. Further, over the past decade, the number of uninsured increased by 54% in households earning between $50,000 and $75,000 and by 130% among households earning $75,000 or more. By contrast, in households earning less than $50,000 the number of uninsured decreased approximately 3% [12].

These results are contrary to the normal expectation of economists. Economic theory teaches that as people earn higher incomes, they should be more willing to purchase insurance to protect their income against claims arising from expensive medical bills.

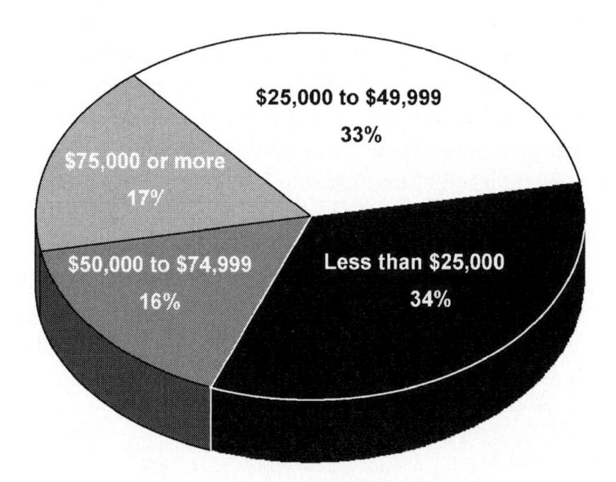

Fig. 1. Income distribution of the uninsured, 2003. (*From* DeNavas-Walt C, Proctor BD, Mills RJ. Income, poverty, and health insurance coverage in the United States: 2003. Current Population Reports, Consumer Income P60–226. Washington (DC): US Census Bureau, US Government Printing Office; 2004.)

Similarly, as people become wealthier the value of insuring against wealth depletion (eg, by a catastrophic illness) also rises. Insurance should be positively correlated with income and wealth accumulation. The fact that the number of uninsured rose over the past decade while incomes were rising and that the greatest increase was among higher-income families suggests that something else is happening to make insurance less attractive.

Some information about middle-class families who are voluntarily uninsured is provided by a California survey of the uninsured with incomes of more than 200% of poverty [13]. Forty percent owned their own homes and more than half owned a personal computer. Twenty percent worked for an employer that offered health benefits, but half of those declined coverage for which they were eligible. This group was not opposed to insurance in general, however, because 90% had purchased auto, home, or life insurance in the past.

The existence of voluntary uninsurance raises a profound public policy question. Economists assume that if people choose A rather than B they are revealing through their actions that they prefer A to B. Further, if people act in accordance with their preferences one is entitled to say they are better off from their own point of view.

From the economist's perspective, the case for doing something about the uninsured rests on its effects on people other than the uninsured. External effects, as shown below, are quite substantial; but if the goal of the reform is to minimize external costs for others, the reform looks quite different from a reform that focuses on the uninsured.

Policy proposals

A number of proposals seek to reduce or eliminate the problem of uninsurance. For example, Physicians for a National Health Program proposes a system of taxpayer-funded, free health care, making government the universal insurer of everyone [14]. Both major candidates in the 2004 presidential campaign proposed offering tax subsidies for private insurance, to individuals and to employers. All of these proposals are highly expensive relative to any reasonable estimate of their probability of success in insuring the uninsured. For example, the National Center for Policy Analysis estimated that Senator John Kerry's plan would have cost just over $1 trillion over 10 years [15]. An American Enterprise Institute study placed the cost of the Kerry plan at $1.5 trillion and President Bush's plan at $128.6 billion. This results in a cost of $1919 per newly insured individual for the Bush plan (almost $8000 for a family of four) and $5494 for the Kerry plan (almost $22,000 for a family of four). Using the candidates' own figures, the Bush plan would have cost $1667 per newly insured, whereas the Kerry plan would have cost about double that amount [16,17].

A different approach is to require individuals to purchase insurance (much as it is now required that people who drive a car have a driver's license) or to require employers to insure their own employees. Proposals to impose mandates on the private sector typically offer a pay-or-play option: either provide insurance or pay a sum of money to the government and let the government handle the problem. There are many problems with mandates, but the most important problem is this: with a pay-or-play approach, no mandate is actually needed.

To the advocates of mandates, the question can always be asked: What are you going to do with people who disobey the mandate? As a practical matter, no one is suggesting that they be put in jail. One is left with imposing a financial penalty (eg, a fine). But a system that fines people who are uninsured ipso facto is indistinguishable from a system that subsidizes those who insure, the subsidy being the absence of the fine. That is the system already in place.

Reasons for uninsurance

Although most people in health policy believe that the existence of millions of uninsured people is a major public policy problem, politicians at both the state and federal level are reflecting voter indifference through their failure to act. The probable reason for this indifference is that uninsured families discover how to get health care even if they have no insurance. They do so in one of two ways: they manage to get insurance after they get sick or they manage to get free care.

A proliferation of state laws has made it increasingly easy for people to obtain insurance after they get sick. Guaranteed issue regulations (requiring insurers to take all comers, regardless of health status) and community-rating regulations (requiring insurers to charge the same premium to all enrollees, regardless of health status) are a free rider's heaven. They encourage everyone to remain uninsured while healthy, confident that they will always be able to obtain insurance once they get sick. Moreover, as healthy people respond to these incentives by electing to be uninsured, the premium that must be charged to cover costs for those who remain in insurance pools rises. These higher premiums, in turn, encourage even more healthy people to drop their coverage.

Federal legislation has also made it increasingly easy to obtain insurance after one gets sick. The Health Insurance Portability and Accountability Act of 1996 had a noble intent: to guarantee that people who have been paying premiums into the private insurance system do not lose coverage simply because they change jobs. A side effect of pursuing this desirable goal is a provision that allows any small business to obtain insurance regardless of the health status of its employees. This means that a small, mom-and-pop operation can save money by remaining uninsured until a family member gets sick. Individuals can also opt out of their employer's plan and re-enroll after they get sick (they are entitled to full coverage for a preexisting condition after an 18-month waiting period). A group health plan can apply preexisting condition exclusions for no more than 12 months except in the case of late enrollees to whom exclusions can apply for 18 months.

The other lure is the existence of free care for those who cannot or do not pay their medical bills. Although no one knows what the exact number is, public and private spending on free care is considerable. A study by the Texas State Comptroller's office found that Texas spent about $1000 per year on free care for every uninsured person in the state, on the average (Fig. 2) [18]. A less comprehensive, but nonetheless nationwide, study by the Urban Institute estimated that in 2001 the uninsured received nearly $90 billion in care, of which more than one third was uncompensated charity care. Charity care by this calculation was equal to about $767 per uninsured individual. If uncompensated physician care is included (as it was in the Texas study), the total likely approaches $1000 [19].

The Texas estimate is almost 7 years old, and at an annual (health care) rate of inflation of 10%, spending doubles every 7 years. Assuming a more conservative increase of 50% puts spending on the uninsured at almost $1500 per person, or about $6000 a year for a family of four.

Interestingly, $6000 is a sum adequate to purchase private health insurance for a family in most Texas cities. One way to look at the choice many Texas families face is: they can rely on $6000 in free care (on the average) or they can purchase a $6000 private insurance policy with after tax income. Granted, the two alternatives are not exactly comparable. Families surely have more options if they have private insurance. To many, however, the free care alternative seems more attractive.

Rationale for government

Aside from the burden of providing charity care to the poor, is there any legitimate reason for government to care whether people have health insurance? Although many reasons have been offered, the main and by far the most persuasive is the "free rider" argument. According to this argument, health insurance has social benefits, over and above the personal benefits to the person who chooses to insure. The reason is that people who fail to insure are likely to get health care anyway, even if they cannot pay for it,

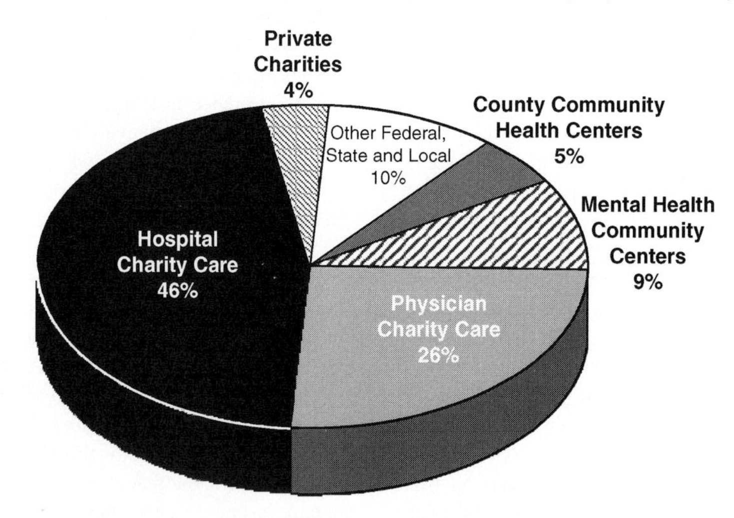

Fig. 2. Health spending on the uninsured in Texas. (*From* Estimated Texas health care spending on the uninsured. Austin (TX): Texas Comptroller's Office, Texas Comptroller of Public Accounts; 2000.)

because the rest of the community is unwilling to allow the uninsured to go without health care, even if their lack of insurance is willful and negligent.

This set of circumstances creates opportunities for some people to be free riders on other people's generosity. In particular, free riders can choose not to pay insurance premiums and to spend the money on other consumption instead, confident that the community as a whole will provide them with care even if they cannot pay for it when it is needed. Being a free rider works because there is a tacit community agreement that no one will be allowed to go without health care. This tacit agreement is so established that it operates as a social contract that many people substitute for a private insurance contract.

A proposal for reform

Fortunately, the concerns of the free rider argument can be met without the disadvantage of other reform proposals. There can be a system that provides a reasonable form of universal coverage for everyone without spending more money and without intrusive and unenforceable government mandates.

Changing the tax system

Currently, the federal government spends more than $189 billion a year on tax subsidies for private insurance [20]. The bulk of these subsidies arise from the fact that employer payments for employee health care are excluded from taxable employee income. Because state tax laws tend to piggyback on the federal tax system, these employer payments avoid state income and payroll taxes. Consider a middle-income family facing a 25% federal income tax rate; a (employer and employee combined) payroll tax rate of 15.3%; and a state income tax of, say, 4%, 5%, or 6%. The ability to exclude employer-paid premiums from taxation means that government is paying almost half the cost of the family's insurance.

These generous tax subsidies undoubtedly encourage people who would otherwise be uninsured to obtain employer-provided insurance. There are three problems, however, with these tax subsidies the way

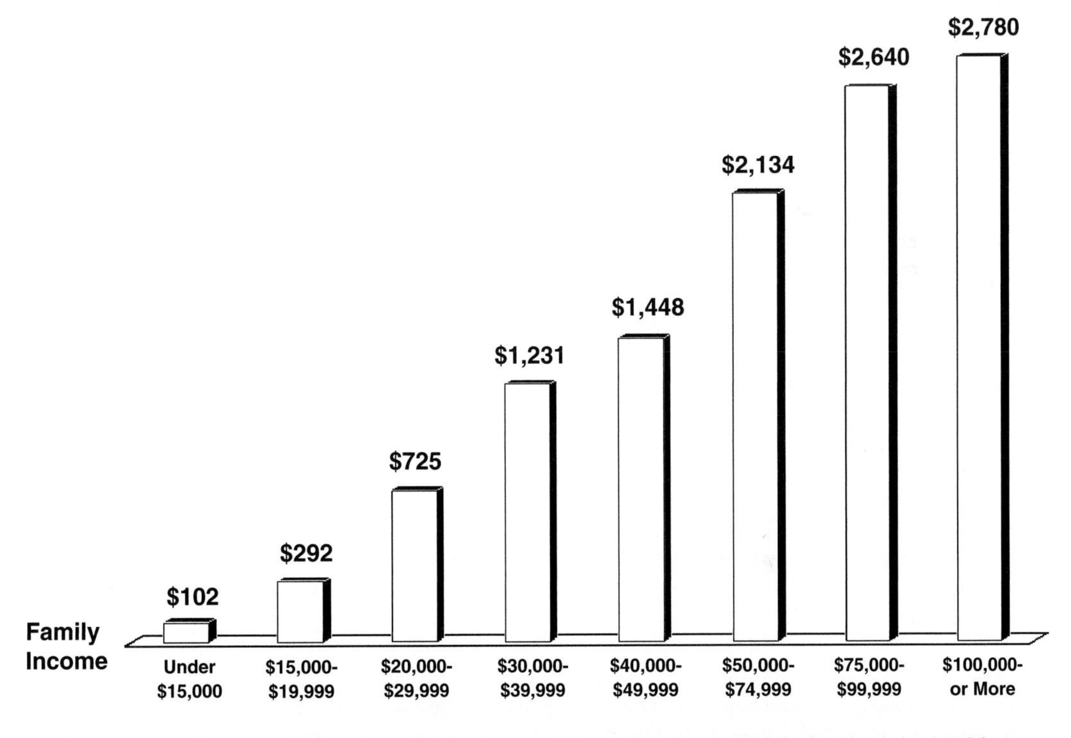

Fig. 3. Average tax subsidy for families, 2004. Lewin Group estimates using the Health Benefits Simulation Model. Average per family is $1482. Includes subsidy from the income tax exclusion, the Social Security income tax exclusion, and the health expenses deduction. (*From* Sheils J, Haught R. The cost of tax-exempt health benefits in 2004. Health Aff (Millwood) Web Exclusive, February 25, 2004. Available at http://content.healthaffairs.org/cgi/reprint/hlthaff.w4.106v1. Accessed July 24, 2005.)

they are structured: (1) the largest subsidies are given to people who need them least; (2) the subsidies are generally not available to most of the uninsured; and (3) the penalties for being uninsured do not fund safety net care.

Under the current system, families who obtain insurance through an employer obtain a tax subsidy worth about $1482 on the average [20]. Not everyone, however, gets the average tax subsidy. Households earning more than $100,000 per year receive an average subsidy of $2780. By contrast, those earning between $20,000 and $30,000 receive only $725 (Fig. 3). One reason is that those earning higher incomes are in higher tax brackets. For example, a family in the 40% tax bracket gets a subsidy of 40 cents for every dollar spent on their health insurance. By contrast, a family in the 15% bracket (paying only the FICA payroll tax) gets a subsidy of only 15 cents on the dollar.

The second problem is that people who do not obtain insurance through an employer get virtually no tax relief if they purchase insurance. Individuals paying out-of-pocket for health care can deduct costs in excess of 7.5% of adjusted gross income. For instance, a family with $50,000 in income is not able to deduct the first $3750 in medical expenses [21]. This means that a middle-income family buying insurance directly must pay almost twice as much after taxes as a similarly situated family whose employer is able to buy the same insurance with pretax dollars. Because most of the uninsured are in this situation, small wonder that reliance on a (free care) safety net looms as an attractive alternative.

Because an uninsured family with an average income does not get a tax subsidy, the family pays about $1482 more in taxes than families that have employer-provided insurance. Instead of describing the current system as one that subsidizes employer-provided insurance, it could, with equal validity, be described as one that penalizes the lack of employer-provided insurance.

Any incentive system can be described in one of two ways: as a system that grants subsidies to those who insure and withholds them from those who do not; or as a system that penalizes the uninsured and refrains from penalizing the insured. Either description is valid, because a subsidy is simply the mirror image of a penalty.

Under the current system the uninsured pay higher taxes because they do not enjoy the tax relief given to those who have employer-provided insurance. These higher taxes are a "fine" for being uninsured. The problem is that the extra taxes paid are simply lumped in with other revenues collected by the US Treasury Department, whereas the expense of delivering free care falls to local doctors and hospitals.

How can these defects be corrected? First, a uniform, refundable tax credit should be offered to every individual for the purchase of private insurance. The Bush administration has proposed a $1000 per person refundable tax credit, or $3000 per family. This tax credit phases out as income rises, however, and virtually vanishes when family income reaches about $80,000 (the author helped formulate the administration's proposal). In general, social interest in whether someone is insured is largely independent of income. In general, a $100,000-a-year family can generate hospital bills it cannot pay almost as easily as a $30,000-a-year family. One can readily grant that there is no social reason to care whether Bill Gates is insured. There could be an income or wealth threshold, beyond which the subsidy-penalty system does not apply. As a practical matter, however, there are so few individuals who would qualify for an exemption that uniform treatment for everyone is administratively attractive. For this reason and practical considerations, the tax credit should be independent of income. Second, all forms of private insurance should be subsidized at the same rate. There is no socially good reason why individuals who cannot obtain insurance through an employer should be penalized when they buy insurance on their own. Third, the higher taxes paid by people who turn down the offer of the tax credit (and through that act elect to be uninsured) should flow to local communities where the uninsured live to be available to pay for care that uninsured patients cannot afford to pay on their own.

Changing the Social Security net

The problem with the current system of spending subsidies is that they encourage people to be uninsured. Why pay for expensive private health insurance when free care provided through public programs is de facto insurance? Think of the system that provides free health care services as "safety net insurance," and note that reliance on the safety net is not as valuable to patients as ordinary private insurance, other things equal. The privately insured patient has more choices of doctors and hospital facilities. Further, safety net care is probably much less efficient (eg, using emergency rooms to provide care that is more economic in a free-standing clinic). As a result, per dollar spent the privately insured patient probably gets more care and better care. It is in society's interest not to encourage people to be in the public sector rather than the private sector.

To avert the perverse incentives the current system creates, people who rely on the free care system should be able to apply those dollars instead to the purchase of private insurance and the accompanying private health care that private insurance makes possible. A mechanism for accomplishing this result follows.

Integrating taxing and spending decisions

Let us now put the pieces together [22,23]. Under an ideal system, the government offers every individual a subsidy. If the individual obtained private insurance, the subsidy is realized in the form of lower taxes (in the form of a tax credit). Alternatively, if the individual chose to be uninsured, the subsidy is sent to a safety net agency in the community where the individual lives (Fig. 4).

The uniform subsidy should reflect the value society places on having one more person insured. But what is that value? An empirically verifiable number is at hand, so long as one is willing to accept the political system as dispositive. It is the amount one expects to spend (from public and private sources) on free care for that person when he or she is uninsured. For example, if society is spending $1500 per year on free care for the uninsured, on the average, one should be willing to offer $1500 to everyone who obtains private insurance. Failure to subsidize private insurance as generously as free care is subsidized encourages people to choose the latter over the former.

One way to think of such an arrangement is to see it as a system under which the uninsured as a group pay for their own free care. That is, in the very act of turning down a tax credit (by choosing not to insure) uninsured individuals pay extra taxes equal to the average amount of free care given annually to the uninsured (Fig. 5).

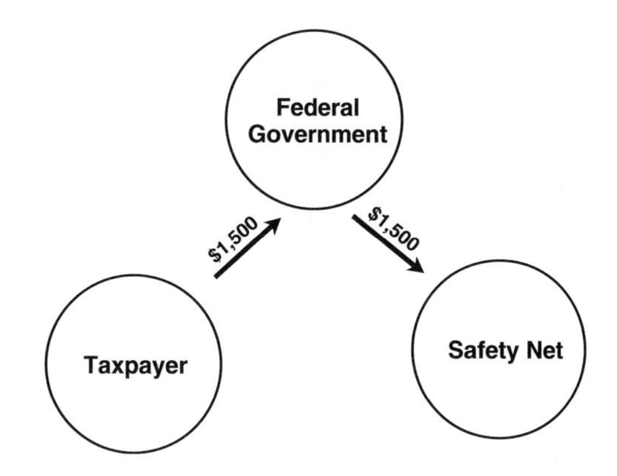

Fig. 5. The marginal effect of choosing to be uninsured.

How can the subsidies for those who choose to move from being uninsured to insured be funded? By reversing the process: at the margin, the subsidy should be funded by the reduction in expected free care that person would have consumed if uninsured. Suppose everyone in Dallas County chose to obtain private insurance, relying on a refundable $1500 federal income tax credit to pay the premiums. As a result, Dallas County no longer needs to spend $1500 per person on the uninsured. All of the money that previously funded safety net medical care could be used to fund the private insurance premiums (Fig. 6).

In this way, people who leave the social safety net and obtain private insurance actually furnish the funding needed to pay their private insurance premiums, at least at the margin. They do this by allowing public authorities to reduce safety net spending by an amount equal to the private insurance tax subsidy. Some patients may be high cost. In a private insurance market, insurers do not agree to insure someone for $1000 if his or her expected cost

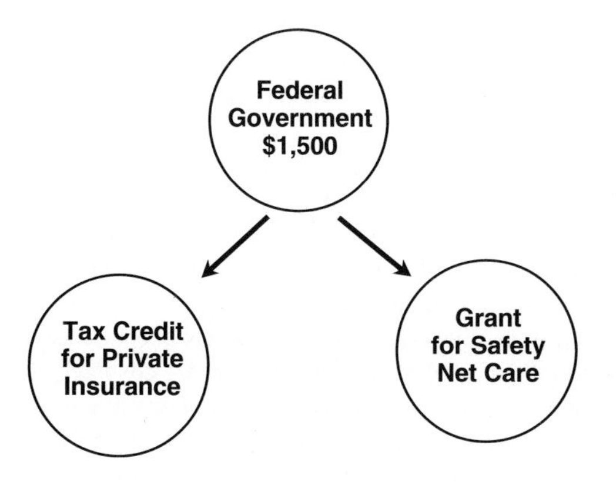

Fig. 4. The $1500 federal guarantee.

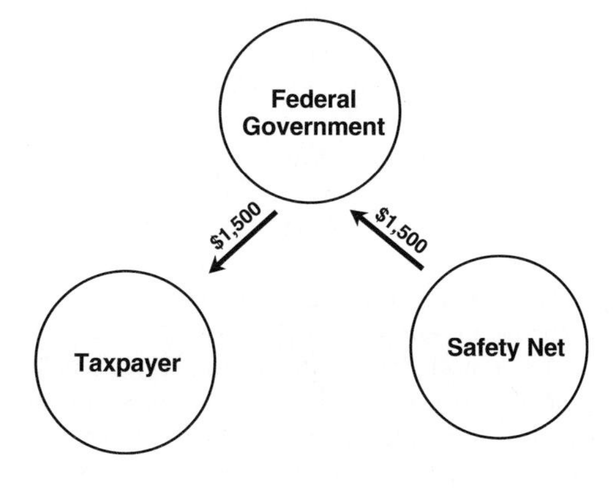

Fig. 6. The marginal effect of choosing to be insured.

of care is, say, $5000. But if the safety net agency expects a $5000 savings as a result of the loss of a patient to a private insurer, the agency should be willing to pay up to $5000 to subsidize the private insurance premium. The additional, higher subsidy could be incorporated into the tax credit or added as a supplement to the tax credit.

Implementing reform

How can this scheme be implemented? To implement the program, all the federal government needs to know is how many people live in each community. In principle, it is offering each of them an annual $1500 tax credit. Some will claim the full credit. Some will claim a partial credit (because they will only be insured for part of a year). Others will claim no credit. What the government pledges to each community is $1500 times the number of people. The portion of this sum that is not claimed on tax returns should be available as block grants to be spent on indigent health care.

How does the federal government manage to reduce safety net spending when uninsured people elected to obtain private insurance? Because much of the safety net expenditure already consists of federal funds, the federal government could use its share to fund private insurance tax credits instead. For the remainder, the federal government could reduce block grants to states for Medicaid and other programs.

Advantages of reform

The goal of health insurance reform is not to get everyone insured (indeed, everyone is already in a loose sense insured). Instead, the goal is to reach a point at which there is societal indifference about whether one more person obtains private insurance as an alternative to relying on the social safety net. That is the point at which the marginal cost (in terms of subsidy) to the remaining members of society of the last person induced to insure is equal to the marginal benefit to the remaining members of society (in terms of the reduction in cost of free care). Once this condition is satisfied, it follows that the number of people who remain uninsured is optimal, and that number is not zero.

This is achieved by taking the average amount spent on free care and making it available for the purchase of private insurance. In the previous example, the government guarantees that $1500 is available, depending on the choice of insurance system. From a policy perspective, there is indifference about the choice people make.

A common misconception is that health insurance reform costs money. For example, if health insurance for 40 million people costs $1500 a person, some conclude that the government needs to spend an additional $65 billion a year to get the job done. What this conclusion overlooks is that $65 billion or more is already being spent on free care for the uninsured, and if all 40 million uninsured suddenly became insured they would free up the $65 billion from the social safety net.

At nearly $2 trillion dollars a year [24], there is no reason to believe the health care system is spending too little money. To the contrary, attempting to insure the uninsured by spending more money has the perverse effect of contributing to health care inflation. Getting all the incentives right may involve shifting around a lot of money (ie, reducing subsidies that are currently too large and increasing subsidies that are too small.) It may also mean making some portion of people's tax liability contingent on proof of insurance [25]. It need not add to budgetary outlays.

There is virtually nothing in the tax code about what features a health insurance plan must have to qualify for a tax subsidy. The exceptions are mandated maternity coverage and coverage of a 48-hour hospital stay after a well-baby delivery if requested by a patient and physician. Insurance purchased commercially, around two thirds of the total, is regulated by the state governments. But the federal tax subsidy applies to whatever plans state governments allow to be sold [26]. In this sense, the federal role is strictly financial. That is, the current tax break is based solely on the number of dollars taxpayers spend on health insurance, not on the features of the health plans themselves.

This practice is sensible and should be continued. Aside from an interest in encouraging catastrophic insurance, there is no social reason why government at any level should dictate the content of health insurance plans. To continue the example, the role of the federal government should be to ensure that $1500 is available. It should leave the particulars of the insurance contract to the market, and it should leave decisions about how to operate the safety net health care to local citizens and their elected representatives.

Under the current system, when people lose or drop their employer-provided insurance coverage, the federal government receives more in taxes as a result. But it makes no extra contribution to any local health care safety net. As a consequence, the growth in the uninsured is straining the finances of many urban hospitals. The problem is exacerbated by less generous federal reimbursement for Medicaid and Medicare and by increasing competitiveness in the hospital sector. Traditionally, hospitals have covered losses that arise from people who cannot pay for their care by overcharging those who can pay. But as the market becomes more competitive, these overcharges are shrinking. There is no such thing as "cost shifting" in a competitive market.

Under this proposal, there is a guaranteed, steadily stream of funds available to local communities who provide indigent care. The funding expands and contracts as the number of uninsured expands and contracts.

Summary

Reform of the United States health care system is less complicated than at first might appear. The building blocks of an ideal system are already in place. The federal government already generously subsidizes private health insurance and safety net care. What is wrong with the current system is that there are too many perverse incentives.

One could reasonably argue that government is doing more harm than good, and that a laissez faire policy is better than what is now in place. Nonetheless, if government is going to be involved in a major way in the health care system, perverse incentives should be replaced with neutral ones. At a minimum, government policy should be neutral between private insurance and the social safety net, never spending more on free care for the uninsured than it spends to encourage the purchase of private insurance. Careful application of this principle would go a long way toward creating an ideal health care system.

References

[1] DeNavas-Walt C, Proctor BD, Mills RJ. Income, poverty, and health insurance coverage in the United States: 2003. Current Population Reports, Consumer Income P60–226. Washington (DC): US Census Bureau, US Government Printing Office; 2004.

[2] Nelson L. How many people lack health insurance and for how long? Congressional Budget Office, May 2003. Available at: http://www.cbo.gov/showdoc.cfm?index=4210&sequence=0. Accessed July 25, 2005.

[3] Alonso-Zaldivar SR. Number of uninsured may be overstated, studies suggest. Los Angeles Times April 26, 2005;Part A:14.

[4] Mills RJ, Bhandari S. Health insurance coverage in the United States: 2002. Current Population Reports, P60–223. Washington (DC): US Census Bureau, US Government Printing Office; 2003.

[5] Marquis S, Long SH. The uninsured access gap: narrowing the estimates. Inquiry 1994–1995;31:405–14.

[6] Marquis S, Long SH. The uninsured access gap and the cost of universal coverage. Health Aff (Millwood) 1994;13:11–20.

[7] Davidoff A, Garrett B, Yemane A. Medicaid-eligible adults who are not enrolled: who are they and do they get the care they need? Urban Institute, Series A, No. A-48: Washington (DC): Urban Institute; 2002.

[8] Dubay L, Haley J, Kenney G. Children's eligibility for Medicaid and SCHIP: a view from 2000. Urban Institute, Series B, No. B-41: Washington (DC): Urban Institute; 2002.

[9] The uninsured in America. Lanham (MD): Blue Cross Blue Shield Association; 2003.

[10] Goodman J, Musgrave G, Herrick D. Lives at risk: single payer national health insurance around the world. Lanham (MD): Rowman and Littlefield; 2004.

[11] Cunningham PJ, Schaefer E, Hogan C. Who declines employer-sponsored health insurance and is uninsured? Issue Brief No. 22. Washington (DC): Center for Studying Health System Change; 1999.

[12] Herrick DM. Is there a crisis of the uninsured? Brief Analysis No. 484. Dallas (TX): National Center for Policy Analysis; 2004.

[13] Yegian JM, Pockell DG, Smith MD, et al. The nonpoor uninsured in California, 1998. Health Aff (Millwood) 2000;19:58–64.

[14] Physicians' Working Group on Single-Payer National Health Insurance. Proposal for health care reform. Chicago: Physicians for a National Health Program; 2001.

[15] Goodman JC, Herrick DM. The case against John Kerry's health plan. NCPA Policy Report No. 269. Dallas (TX): National Center for Policy Analysis; 2004.

[16] Antos J, King R, Wildsmith T. Analyzing the Kerry and Bush health proposals: estimates of cost and impact. Washington (DC): American Enterprise Institute; 2004.

[17] Herrick DM. Bush versus Kerry on health care. Brief Analysis No. 468. Dallas (TX): National Center for Policy Analysis; 2004.

[18] Texas estimated health care spending on the uninsured. Austin (TX): Texas Comptroller of Public Accounts; 1999.

[19] Hadley J, Holahan J. How much medical care do the uninsured use, and who pays for it? Health Aff (Millwood) 2003. Available at: http://content.healthaffairs.org/cgi/reprint/hlthaff.w3.66v1. Accessed July 25, 2005.

[20] Sheils J, Haught R. The cost of tax-exempt health benefits in 2004. Health Aff (Millwood) 2004. http://content.healthaffairs.org/cgi/reprint/hlthaff.w4.106v1. Accessed July 25, 2005.

[21] Topic 502 Medical and Dental Expenses, Internal Revenue Service, US Department of the Treasury. Available at: www.irs.gov/taxtopics/tc502.html. Accessed July 25, 2005.

[22] Goodman JC, Musgrave GL. Patient power: solving

America's health care crisis. Washington: Cato Institute; 1992.
[23] Etheredge L. A flexible benefits tax credit for health insurance and more. Health Aff (Millwood). Available at: http://content.healthaffairs.org/cgi/reprint/hlthaff.w1.1v1. Accessed July 25, 2005.
[24] Heffler S, Smith S, Keehan S, et al. US health spending projections for 2004–2014. Health Aff (Millwood) 2005. Available at: http://content.healthaffairs.org/cgi/reprint/hlthaff.w5.74v1. Accessed July 25, 2005.
[25] Steuerle CE. Child credits: opportunity at the door. Washington (DC): Urban Institute; 1997.
[26] Marquis MS, Long SH. Recent trends in self-insured employer health plans. Health Aff (Millwood) 1999; 18:161–6.

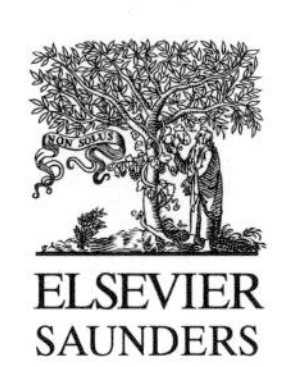

ELSEVIER
SAUNDERS

Thorac Surg Clin 15 (2005) 513 – 518

THORACIC
SURGERY
CLINICS

Compliance with HIPAA Regulations: Ethics and Excesses

Peter Angelos, MD, PhD

Department of Surgery, Northwestern University, Feinberg School of Medicine, 201 East Huron Street, NMH/Galter, Room 10-105, Chicago, IL 60611, USA

On April 14, 2003, regulations developed by the US Department of Health and Human Services designed to give patients more control over their personal health information first took effect. These regulations were promulgated in response to the Health Insurance Portability and Accountability Act of 1996 (HIPAA), which Congress passed after calling on the Department of Health and Human Services to issue privacy protections. The goal of the HIPAA regulations was to:

> Ensure a national floor of privacy protections for patients by limiting the ways that health plans, pharmacies, hospitals and other covered entities can use patients' personal medical information. The regulations protect medical records and other individually identifiable health information, whether it is on paper, in computers or communicated orally [1].

These regulations made explicit certain requirements for health plans, pharmacies, doctors, and other covered entities to maintain the confidentiality of protected health information about their patients.

Taken at face value, the HIPAA regulations seemed to provide important safeguards for patients. Certainly, no one could argue that it was a bad thing to prevent doctors or health plans from using patient information for marketing or that problems would be created if doctors were required to ensure that their communications with patients were kept confidential. In the months before and immediately after HIPAA regulations took effect, however, many assumptions were made and myths created about what physicians and other medical personnel were allowed to do with respect to communicating with patients. In fact, a whole cottage industry of HIPAA compliance arose designed to allow physicians and medical institutions to meet the letter of the law and thereby avoid the dreaded possibility of financial sanctions. This article explores some of the important ways that HIPAA regulations were thought to affect the interactions of surgeons and patients. Considered are some cases where possible problems were encountered, and whether the problems are actual or purely imagined. The HIPAA regulations are considered with a modicum of common sense and professional judgment. Also explored are some real ethical issues that HIPAA regulations do raise, especially when it comes to medical research.

Goals of regulations

The primary goal of the HIPAA regulations was to protect the confidentiality of patient information in the era of electronic health care transactions [2]. Privacy generally has been taken to mean the "right to be left alone" [3]. Although privacy may specifically refer to informational privacy [4], usually the term "confidentiality" is used to refer to the importance of keeping information about patients from disclosure to third parties. As Moskop and colleagues [2] have pointed out, it is interesting to note that although the two distinct concepts of privacy and confidentiality are the bases of the regulations, there are few references to confidentiality in the regulations. In fact, HIPAA is frequently referred to as the "HIPAA privacy rule."

The admonition to maintain the confidences of patients is one of the well-known tenets of the Hippocratic Oath. As such, there is little need to spend time

E-mail address: pangelos@nmff.org

1547-4127/05/$ – see front matter
doi:10.1016/j.thorsurg.2005.06.006

deriving the importance of this principle of medical ethics. In an era of large health care institutions in which confidential information about patients is transferred electronically on a regular basis, one can readily imagine the increased risks of breeches of confidentiality. The HIPAA regulations were an attempt to make clear to health care providers that respecting the privacy of confidential information was not just a good thing to do for ethical patient care, but in fact it was required by law. The regulations set out possible civil and criminal penalties for violations of the HIPAA regulations.

As with any legal requirement, there are clear exceptions to the prohibition of disclosing personal health information without the patient's written authorization [2]:

1. Personal health information may be given to the patient himself or herself.
2. Caregivers may use and disclose personal health information for their own treatment, payment, and health care operations activities (eg, quality assessment, education of health care professionals, insurance underwriting, and business management).
3. With the patient's "informal permission," caregivers may disclose personal health information to family members or in facility directories.
4. Caregivers may use and disclose personal health information for 12 "national priority purposes."

The national priority purposes include [5]:

1. When required by law
2. For public health activities
3. For reporting of abuse, neglect, or domestic violence
4. For health oversight activities
5. For judicial and administrative proceedings
6. For law enforcement purposes
7. For disclosures about deceased persons to coroners, medical examiners, and funeral directors
8. For organ, eye, and tissue donation purposes
9. For some types of research
10. To avert a serious threat to the health or safety of a person or the public
11. For specialized government functions, such as military missions or correctional activities
12. For Workman's Compensation claims

Among the national priority purposes listed previously, number 9 refers specifically to research "when an institutional review board has waived the authorization requirement."

Hype about the Health Insurance Portability and Accountability Act regulations

As reasonable as some might have thought the idea of regulations to protect private patient information to be, the actual implementation of the HIPAA regulations created many concerns. First of all, the regulations required hospitals and medical clinics to hold training sessions for providers and to ensure that patients knew about the regulations. These training sessions could have been seen as an important educational opportunity to sharpen the awareness of medical care providers about the need to protect private patient information. Instead, the training sessions often seemed to become bogged down in the minutia of a complex set of regulations and the threat of financial penalties led some institutions to hire legal "HIPAA consultants." Because no one had any idea how the federal government would interpret the regulations, these consultants often counseled physicians and institutions that the strictest possible interpretation of the regulations is the safest approach as far as reducing the risk of possible sanctions.

The HIPAA regulations take up approximately 31 pages of single-spaced, triple-columned text. As a result, there are many legal issues that are raised by the regulations. Nevertheless, much of the concern for individual physicians has focused on the "incidental" disclosures that may occur while providing care to patients. As Lo and colleagues [6] have stated:

> In the course of good patient care, communications among health care workers treating the patient may be seen or overheard by someone else. In addition, physicians may transmit patient information to a family member or friend involved in the patient's care. These uses and disclosures of information are termed *incidental* because they result from or are "incident" to a permitted use or disclosure.

In the following pages, no effort is made to provide a close legal analysis of the regulations. Instead, some of the questions surrounding incidental disclosures are considered by using a series of cases with discussions. There are difficulties when trying to bring legal requirements and ethical principles together. The goal of the following discussion, however, is to suggest that the HIPAA regulations are not really as different from the practices of good medical care as many believe. In addition, how the HIPAA regulations may be beneficial to the ethical practice of medicine by providing a legal framework for much of the ethical practices that have been used for years is explored. Although realizing that something is "required by law" does not make it more ethical, knowing that it is required by law may serve to emphasize why some ethical principles are taken so seriously that they are now backed up by law.

Illustrative cases

The following illustrative cases are designed to raise some of the concerns that surgeons have with the HIPAA regulations. Some of the cases are real and some are fictional; however, all have been suggested by surgeons as raising difficulties that HIPAA either creates or exacerbates for surgical care.

Case 1

A 50-year-old male patient was brought to the emergency room conscious but confused and intoxicated after having been involved in a motor vehicle collision. The patient was an unrestrained passenger. Also brought in was the restrained driver, a young woman, who has only minor injuries. The patient's driver's license indicates that he is from another state. The driver of the vehicle states that she only just met the patient at a bar earlier in the evening and knows nothing about him. During his evaluation, he develops respiratory distress such that he requires emergent intubation. Imaging suggests he has a multiple rib fractures and a pulmonary contusion. The trauma surgery service that is admitting the patient is unsure whether a call should be made to the patient's spouse or whether making such a call might create additional problems. The hospital administrator on call believes that there will be a clear HIPAA violation if the patient's family is notified of the admission without the patient giving consent for this disclosure of information. Without contacting the spouse, however, no surrogate decision maker will have been identified in case consent for a procedure is needed.

This case describes the type of emergency situation that is commonly faced by surgeons. Clearly, regardless of HIPAA regulations, there is an ethical issue of whether or not to notify the family of this admission. What is often difficult for the treating physicians to know is whether HIPAA regulations provide any assistance in a case such as this, or if the regulations only add the stress of sanctions if the physicians act contrary to the regulations. In fact, the HIPAA Privacy Rule does permit sharing of "information that is directly relevant to the involvement of a spouse, family members, friends, or other persons identified by the patient, in the patient's care" [7]. If in the judgment of the treating physician the disclosure to family is in the patient's best interests, even without the patient's approval, the trauma surgeons should notify the spouse. As Lo and colleagues [6] have emphasized, it is important to realize that HIPAA regulations encourage the exercise of professional judgment to determine what is in the patient's best interests if the patient is not able to make his or her wishes known.

Consider if this case were changed slightly. Instead of the situation as described where the patient made no wishes known, what if in the short time between entering the emergency department and his intubation the patient repeatedly stated that no one is to call his family? In this situation, with information that the patient has objected to the disclosure of information to the family, the trauma surgeons should not proceed to notify the spouse. In this new situation, the HIPAA privacy rule provides guidance that the patient's wishes regarding limiting disclosure of information even to families should be respected. Based on the importance of exercise of professional judgment noted previously, however, if the patient were not able to be extubated for many days, the situation might arise where the physician's judgment of the patient's best interest would allow for contacting the family. In this scenario, the HIPAA regulations provide no specific guidance, yet if such a decision is made by the physicians in a careful and deliberate manner, the risks of penalties based on HIPAA seem low. Certainly, the considerations that might lead the physicians to come to a decision that it is necessary to contact the spouse should be well-documented in the medical record.

Consider if the patient were brought in unconscious and alone with no emergency contact information. According to the HIPAA privacy rules, could the physicians caring for the patient transmit confidential medical information to the police department to try to contact the family? Despite the limitations on such communication that many had assumed HIPAA would require, such information disclosure is clearly allowed because it is in the best interests of the patient. In such a situation, the information that is transmitted should be limited to the minimum necessary to allow identification of the patient's family.

Case 2

A patient has undergone a video-assisted thoracoscopic resection of a pulmonary nodule. The patient has just been extubated after the successful completion of the procedure. The surgeon is paged to the family waiting room with the message that a large number of family members are waiting for her arrival to discuss the outcome of the operation. Although such discussion had been routine before HIPAA regulations going into effect, the surgeon hesitates because she had been told by colleagues that HIPAA prohibited such discussions without the patient's prior written approval.

This simple case illustrates some of the problems with the hype that surrounded HIPAA regulations going into effect. Unfortunately, much erroneous information was informally communicated among health care providers about what was allowed and what was prohibited under HIPAA. Such disclosure of the successful outcome of the procedure is clearly allowed to persons accompanying the patient to the hospital [7]. HIPAA regulations do push physicians to be careful, however, about what information is provided. If the patient in Case 2 had been asked before surgery, "Is there anyone in the waiting room that I should talk to after the surgery"? and the patient had answered, "No," then a request to speak to family members in the waiting room should be more carefully considered. The surgeon should ensure that she knows who she is speaking with and the relationship of that person to the patient. One certainly does not want to provide information to a reporter about a patient whose operation is newsworthy. The surgeon is wise to limit such communication to the very basic information rather than a detailed discussion of the pathology report, further treatment options, and so forth. The benefit of HIPAA regulations in such situations is that if a patient requests that no information be conveyed to family members, then the surgeon has clear regulatory support for maintaining such confidences.

Case 3

A 78-year-old woman has been in the surgical ICU for several weeks after complications following coronary artery bypass surgery. The patient has suffered a stroke and has developed renal failure, pancreatitis, pneumonia, and an upper gastrointestinal hemorrhage. Several different services including neurology, nephrology, infectious disease, gastroenterology, and general surgery have been consulted. The patient's family is concerned about the large numbers of attending physicians, fellows, residents, and medical students from these various services that have been consulted who are all seeing her and discussing her condition in the surgical ICU conference room. The family is upset about the complications and announces to the nurses that, "Based on HIPAA, no one but those care-givers that have been approved by the patient or family are allowed to receive private medical information about the patient." The managing cardiac surgeon is unsure how to respond to this ultimatum.

In this case, we are presented with one of the limits of the patient or family's control over information about a patient. The Department of Health and Human Services web site on frequently asked questions makes clear that doctors and other providers may share patient health information for treatment without the patient's authorization [7]. It is essential that physicians and other health care providers understand that the HIPAA regulations have been set up with the clear goal that protecting private information should not interfere with providing good medical care. Patients cannot invoke HIPAA regulations to limit consultations of other health care providers to help manage the patient's numerous problems. From an ethical point of view, however, this statement by the family is a clear indication that communication between the managing surgeon and the family has not been ideal. Even in the face of complications and the disappointments that families may have about the outcome of a particular operation, attention should be directed to addressing the family's concerns so that they understand why the multiple consultants are in the patient's best interests. The medical providers should be careful not to use the fact that HIPAA does not require families to give consent for medically necessary consultations to lessen the importance of communicating clearly with the family about the patient's condition and what is being done to address it.

In Case 3, the importance of medically necessary consultants to the patient's outcome is clear. What about the request, however, that neither medical students nor nursing students interact with the patient? Certainly, one cannot use the argument that, based on HIPAA, the interaction of these students is in the patient's best interests. Although the attention of such individuals may actually prove to be beneficial to the patient, HIPAA allows for the involvement of these students on the basis of the importance of education for the medical profession. There is even specific allowance for student participation in patient care for educational purposes without the patient's written authorization. Such allowance under HIPAA should not lead to a disregard of patient wishes regarding the involvement of students in their care [8]. It is certainly not necessary, however, to obtain written authorization from the patient before communication with students for medical educational purposes. As Moskop and colleagues [8] have pointed out, if the observer in the emergency department is a high school student considering a medical career rather than a medical or nursing student, then explicit consent should be sought from the patient before this person's involvement.

Case 4

After showing a colleague from another institution around the clinic, a director of a large thoracic surgery clinic is told by this colleague that several HIPAA problems were identified. First of all, the colleague points out that the patients should not be asked to sign in when they enter the clinic waiting room because this exposes their names to the view of others. Second, staff should never call out patient's names in the waiting rooms because names are protected information. Third, no information should ever be shared with a patient's other physicians without the patient's written authorization. Although the doctors and nurses in the clinic have been very sensitive not to discuss patient details within earshot of other patients, the director believes that if these other recommendations are all acted on, it is very difficult to maintain the appointment schedule and communicate with referring physicians.

This case addresses a number of issues in the outpatient setting that have been raised by many who have little knowledge about HIPAA regulations. Undoubtedly, HIPAA regulations do add to the administrative burdens in many clinical settings. Patients must be given written notice of how their personal medical information may be used. They must also be asked to sign or otherwise acknowledge that they have received such information. As a result, every new physician office visit or a trip to a new pharmacy to pick up a prescription medication now results in this mandatory transfer of information. The regulations, however, do not require doctors' offices completely to change the way that care is rendered. Although the regulations are designed to raise the level of awareness about the serious ramifications that might occur if private information about patients is disclosed for reasons other than those that benefit the patient's medical well-being, the regulations do specifically allow the communication of medical information among the patient's care providers. The regulations also do not forbid patients to sign in, and do not require that every office hand out pagers so that names do not need to be called out [7]. They do require physicians and medical offices to take "reasonable steps," however, to ensure that their communications with patients are kept confidential. If a patient requests that he or she be called at home and not at work, the physician should comply with that request. Physicians are still allowed to communicate with patients over the telephone and even leave telephone messages, but the nature of the information left on an answering machine, for example, should be carefully considered such that confidential information is limited.

Health Insurance Portability and Accountability Act regulations and research

When it comes to conducting research, HIPAA regulations should be very strictly interpreted. In contrast to the allowance for the use of professional judgment for disclosure of private information that is necessary for good patient care, research by its very nature is not directed specifically at benefiting the individual patient. Any disclosure of private information for research purposes must be preceded by the patient's specific consent, unless the research is exempted from such requirements by an institutional review board. HIPAA specifies that an institutional review board may grant such an exemption from individual authorization if [9]:

1. Its use involves no more than a minimal risk (meaning researchers plan to protect and ultimately destroy identifiers to prevent their reuse)
2. Research could not practicably be conducted without the waiver
3. Research could not practicably be conducted without access to and use of the information

When private information is gathered for research purposes, every attempt should be made to deidentify the information so that individual patients cannot be traced from the research data.

Summary

HIPAA regulations have been seen by many physicians as providing innumerable administrative hoops that require jumping through with no clear benefit for individual patients. Although this article has not comprehensively explored the requirements of HIPAA regulations, it has focused on the issues of "incidental disclosures" that are so important to the daily interactions of physicians and patients. Through the use of illustrative cases, it has been shown that

HIPAA regulations frequently are based on well-accepted ethical principles. Although one should never conclude that changing something from an ethical responsibility to a legal responsibility makes it more important, there is no question that HIPAA regulations have forced physicians to consider more carefully how confidential information may be transmitted to others. As such, physicians should look on HIPAA regulations as largely supporting the use of professional judgment in providing good quality medical care. Although not all aspects of HIPAA are grounded in ethical practices, the overall thrust of the HIPAA regulations is consistent with the ethical practice of medicine and surgery. As a result of this general alignment of the legal and ethical requirements, more attention should be directed by physicians at using good judgment in deciding how to disclose private information, rather than adopting an unreasonable approach that confidentiality may never be breached. As Lo and colleagues [6] have very appropriately pointed out:

> In the context of inadvertent disclosure, the legal risks of good practice are very low. Physicians should work with risk managers and practice administrators to develop policies that promote good communication in patient care, while taking appropriate steps to protect patient privacy.

By adopting such an approach to HIPAA, physicians can abide by the regulations while maintaining high ethical standards and minimizing the impact of the new requirements on physician-patient relationships.

References

[1] United States Department of Health and Human Services Press release Monday April 14, 2003. Available at: http://www.hhs.gov/news. Accessed April 15, 2005.

[2] Moskop JC, Marco CA, Larkin GL, et al. From Hippocrates to HIPAA: privacy and confidentiality in emergency medicine—Part I: conceptual, moral, and legal foundations. Ann Emerg Med 2005;45:53–9.

[3] Warren S, Brandeis L. The right to privacy. Harv Law Rev 1890;4:193–220.

[4] Allen AL. Privacy in health care. In: Reich WT, editor. Encyclopedia of bioethics, vol. 4. New York: Macmillan; 1995. p. 2064–73.

[5] 45 CFR § 164.512.

[6] Lo B, Dornbrand L, Dubler N. HIPAA and patient care: the role for professional judgement. JAMA 2005;293: 1766–71.

[7] Your frequently asked questions on privacy. Available at: http://www.hhs.gov/ocr/hipaa. Accessed April 15, 2005.

[8] Moskop JC, Marco CA, Larkin GL, et al. From Hippocrates to HIPAA: privacy and confidentiality in emergency medicine—Part II: challenges in the emergency department. Ann Emerg Med 2005;45:60–7.

[9] Durham ML. How research will adapt to HIPAA: a view from within the healthcare delivery system. Am J Law Med 2002;28:491–502.

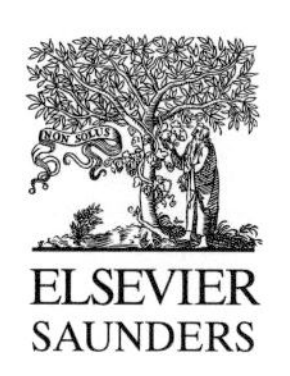

ELSEVIER
SAUNDERS

Thorac Surg Clin 15 (2005) 519 – 525

THORACIC
SURGERY
CLINICS

The Ethics of Living Donor Lung Transplantation

Winfield J. Wells, MD*, Mark L. Barr, MD

Department of Cardiothoracic Surgery, University of Southern California and Childrens Hospital Los Angeles, 4650 Sunset Boulevard, Mailstop #66, Los Angeles, CA 90027, USA

The ethics of living organ donation have been debated since the earliest recognition of the potential advantages of a living donor's organ for transplantation, and the likelihood that living donation could become the preferred approach [1]. Ethical considerations doubled in 1993 when Starnes and colleagues proposed and then performed the first bilateral living donor lobar lung transplantation. Because two living donors are required for the procedure, concerns about the risks of the operation were raised by highly respected bioethicists.

Such opinions and concerns were anticipated and ethical issues had been extensively discussed and were incorporated into the structure of the University of Southern California (USC) living donor lung transplant program, particularly as they pertained to the pretransplant assessment of recipients and donors. This article summarizes the basic concepts and thought processes used in dealing with ethical questions regarding living lung donation.

Traditional medical ethics versus autonomy of the individual

Donation of a pulmonary lobe by a living volunteer is incompatible with the pillar of medical ethics as established by the Hippocratic maxim "primum non nocere" (first do no harm). Although the risk of mortality from donor lobectomy is low, the potential for significant morbidity has been documented in at least two series by experienced transplant teams [2,3]. Because it is not possible to justify a physical benefit to a living donor as implied by "primum non nocere," a more complex set of moral theories has evolved to deal with the realities of advancing transplant therapies.

Beauchamp and Childress [4] have provided a framework for dealing with the complex issues of living organ donation through their four basic principles of biomedical ethics:

1. Respect for autonomy: respecting and accepting the decision-making capacity of the autonomous individual.
2. Nonmaleficence (non nocere): minimizing the causation of harm.
3. Beneficence: providing a benefit and balancing this against risk and cost.
4. Justice: fairly distributing benefits, risks, and costs.

These principles are widely accepted in the biomedical community as a set of practical guidelines that get their roots from elements of more classical utilitarianism, rights- and duty-based theory, and virtue ethics.

Respect for autonomy

Traditional liberal democratic ethical and political thinking hold that an individual is the rightful determinant of his or her actions except when others might be harmed as a result of that action. This implies that people should be allowed to decide what to do with themselves, including making risky choices, if the choices are sufficiently valuable to them.

* Corresponding author.
E-mail address: wwells@chla.usc.edu (W.J. Wells).

1547-4127/05/$ – see front matter
doi:10.1016/j.thorsurg.2005.06.003

Respect for autonomy is a starting point in all bioethical discussion but it must be balanced by medical judgment. This embodies the concept that health professionals may decide against an individual's wishes (ie, living lobar lung donation) when such action is taken for that person's benefit [5]. Medical judgment is based on the ethical principles of beneficence, which balances risks against benefits to provide what is best for the patient. Examples relevant to a potential living lung donor are obvious, such as when the transplant team ensures that a donor is competent to understand the risks of lobectomy and that the donor's judgment is not compromised by developmental delay, illness, or even coercion. Because such compromised individuals are not truly autonomous, there is no moral issue involved in protecting them from potential harm.

The problem of balancing medical judgment against autonomy becomes much more complex when the transplant team must deal with a competent, motivated donor who has significant risk factors (ie, poorly controlled hypertension) for undergoing a major procedure, such as lobectomy. This is a situation of conflicting values and the major question is whether one can assume that the medical team really knows what is in the potential donor's best interest because values are not universally shared. Accepting that living donors have a moral right to take a risk to achieve a substantial benefit for the recipient, and for themselves, the risk must be balanced by the right of health professionals to weigh risk-to-benefit ratio and fit this into acceptable medical practice [5].

When the ethical foundations of living donation were being formulated professional autonomy was taken to empower the transplant team to decide the appropriateness of going forward. The decision, which was based on the group's analysis of risk versus benefit, was made, and given greater weight than that of the donor [6]. In doing this, the ethical principle of nonmaleficence was given special weight, but it was deemed critical that the team not undervalue the potential benefits that might accrue to both the donor and recipient from the living donor organ. Particularly in younger patients, there is the possibility that a pulmonary lobe from a living donor may have an advantage over one from a cadaveric donor [7]. A living lobar lung transplant can be done on relatively short notice in the situation of a recipient who is rapidly deteriorating and would not survive the cadaveric organ waiting list time, which is often greater than a year. A major question regarding lobar lung transplantation that has been unanswered during the last decade has been defining when a potential recipient is too ill to justify placing two healthy donors at risk of donor lobectomy. But despite the high-risk recipient group, this alternative procedure has been life-saving in severely ill patients who would either die or become unsuitable recipients before a cadaveric organ becomes available. The quality of a living donor's lung for transplant is also generally better than that from a cadaveric donor because of the shorter ischemic time and the absence of the sequelae of brain death on various organ systems.

From the perspective of the living donor there are psychologic, emotional, and spiritual benefits in addition to matters of self-esteem, which offset the procedural risks and discomfort, and these must be carefully weighed and not discounted [8]. A better understanding of these issues was an important part of the transition from "living related" to simply a "living" donor lung transplant program in the authors' institution. Early in the experience at USC, donors were always related to the recipient because it was believed that the bond between donor and recipient should be sufficiently close to justify the risk of thoracotomy and lobectomy particularly in the face of an uncertain benefit. Subsequently recognition of the benefits of living donation, both through general information from the transplant community on kidney and liver living donor outcomes and growing experience, loosened the requirement that the donor and recipient be related.

The ethical principles involved in decision making for living organ donors were extensively analyzed by a multidisciplinary group from the transplant community, which included physicians, nurses, psychologists, attorneys, social workers, transplant donors, recipients, and several ethicists. The resulting Consensus Statement on the Live Organ Donor was published in 2000 [9]. It provides a template for the structure of an ethically sound clinical program. Emphasis is placed on ensuring both medical and psychosocial suitability of the potential donor and an optimal informed consent.

Ensuring medical suitability for living lobar transplant is the most easily accomplished of all the tasks in the donor evaluation process. The basic premise is that the donor must be healthy. The program at USC gives consideration to volunteer donors from age 18 to approximately 55 that are preferably no more the 25% above ideal body weight. Donor selection is further based on the results of chest radiograph, pulmonary function testing, ventilation-perfusion scanning, and chest CT scans. Those with a prior smoking history should ideally be tobacco free for at least 6 months and have normal pulmonary function and imaging tests.

For potential donors 40 years of age or more with risk factors for coronary artery disease or with hypertension (which should be well controlled), a cardiac stress test is performed. Echocardiography is also done to rule out significant left ventricular hypertrophy in those with hypertension. Diabetics who are not insulin dependent, have good glycemic control, and show no evidence of end-organ disease have also been considered as potential donors.

This level of careful attention to the medical work-up of potential donors is absolutely essential despite the potentially high cost. The transplant team is ethically bound to make the risk of living donation as low as it can possibly be, and although there have been some serious complications in the living lobar donor cohort in the USC program, among the 289 donors operated from 1993 to the present time there have been no deaths [3].

The psychosocial evaluation of potential donors is among the most important steps in ensuring the ethical grounding of a living donor transplant program, and its importance has been emphasized in the Consensus Statement [9]. A mental health professional that specializes in transplantation issues and is a regular member of the transplant team should carry out this phase of the work-up. This may be a clinical social worker, psychologist, psychiatric nurse specialist, or other similarly trained individual. Ideally the potential living donor has the psychosocial evaluation performed by an independent transplant team member not involved with the recipient, although this may not always be possible.

The most straightforward task in the evaluation is to be sure that the potential donor is competent to make an informed decision by ruling out major uncontrolled psychiatric illness or significant developmental delay. Although a history of mental illness does not automatically preclude living donation, the onus is on the team to be absolutely sure that an individual's problem is stable and well-controlled, as judged by both the donor's treating mental health professional and the transplant team evaluator, who must have the final word.

The psychosocial evaluation must diligently seek out all of the potential causes of mental instability, such as substance abuse, marital discord, or family dysfunction, which might make living donation unacceptably difficult. The possibility of major financial hardship must also be considered and may exclude donation.

In the end, the psychosocial review must ensure that the primary motivation for the living donor is altruism, and that there is absolutely no evidence of coercion. Skillful probing should be able to eliminate such factors as undue family pressure (a fear of being ostracized by the family) if an individual does not come forward as a donor. The possibility that the potential donor is in a subservient position to the recipient must also be eliminated, and guilt should not be a major factor in the decision to donate.

If the psychosocial evaluation uncovers a reluctant donor, the transplant team is in a position to allow the donor to withdraw gracefully from the process. The donor may simply be found to be unsuitable, and there should be no need to provide further explanation because the medical findings are considered to be privileged.

To meet its ethical obligation to a potential living donor the transplant team must obtain a detailed informed consent that provides full disclosure of all possible adverse events. Each step of the process of donation has hazards that must be explained in language that the donor can understand. Even the most highly intelligent individual may not be familiar with medical terms used in clinicians' daily vocabulary. They may be embarrassed to ask what a term as seemingly basic as "hematoma" means.

The risks of the diagnostic procedures and the operation to procure the donated organ (in this case thoracotomy and lobectomy) must be thoroughly explained including the anticipated time to full recovery. Of great importance to most donors is when they can anticipate return to work. Full disclosure also requires that even if there has not been a death or other major complications in a program, these must be mentioned if they are known to have occurred in other transplant centers. The need for follow-up after hospital discharge must also be discussed.

It is important that the disclosure process include an honest and realistic explanation of the expected outcomes for the recipient because most potential living donors are not aware that 5-year survival after lung transplant is in the range of 50% [10]. If the outcomes for a specific program are not as good as those reported from multi-institutional studies, then the program-specific outcomes should be given.

The potential living donor must also be informed of any possible fiscal implications, which could include expenses for travel and lodging, loss of income, or the risk of losing future employment opportunities. The possibility that a history of pulmonary lobectomy might influence the donor's ability to get health, disability, or even life insurance needs to be mentioned.

Finally, similar to the issues involved in psychosocial evaluation, the informed consent should ideally be obtained by someone who has no involvement with the recipient. This person should view himself or herself as an advocate for the potential donor.

Source of donation

At the outset of the living donor experience it was thought that recipients should be listed for cadaveric transplantation because of uncertainties regarding both risks and outcomes. It was also recommended that living donors be directly (genetically) related to the recipient. Compensation of any kind to the donor was considered unacceptable and unethical. Each of these concepts has been challenged and revised, however, as experience has been gained and outcomes documented.

As noted in the World Health Organization resolution on human organ and tissue transplantation, it has been well established for renal transplantation that the living donor provides better tissue for a recipient [11]. When outcomes such as these are documented, it is no longer morally acceptable to require that the option of obtaining a cadaveric organ be exhausted before considering living donors. Potential lung recipients may significantly deteriorate during a waiting period for the living donor operation, increasing their risk, which is ethically unacceptable.

The requirement that living lung donors be related, which was established at the inception of the USC program, was predicated on the idea that the close emotional bond within a family made the risks of thoracotomy and lobectomy more acceptable. Additionally, it was hoped that shared genetic characteristics might improve graft survival. The evidence base, however, does not support this concept. It is now known that kidney transplant graft survival from a spouse or friend (involving a complete HLA mismatch with the recipient) is essentially equal to that from a haploidentical parent or sibling [12]. The same seems to be true for living lobar donor lung transplant. Denying unrelated donors does not seem to be ethically defensible. As this information became known the description of the USC program was changed from "living related lobar lung transplant" to "living donor lobar lung transplant."

To improve the chances of finding a compatible living donor, match exchange programs have been established in several countries [13]. This has allowed living donor organs (kidneys) to be exchanged between pairs of individuals with incompatible ABO blood types or lymphocyte crossmatch. Although some have questioned whether such programs too closely approximate commerce, the majority opinion holds that exchange provides an opportunity that does not otherwise exist in an ethical manner that is in keeping with altruism as the primary donor motivation.

Where there have been exchanges for living kidney donation, each transplant center has made an individual decision about meetings between the donor-recipient pairs. To make the program ethically sound, however, there is an understanding that the recipients and the transplant teams responsible for those individuals must be given full access to information about their potential donor. This allows a fully informed decision about the merits of an exchange.

From a practical standpoint paired living donor exchange programs must schedule the donor operative procedures to be done at the same time to eliminate the possibility that one donor declines at the last moment. The problems surrounding a paired exchange for living lobar lung donation are considerably more complex than that for kidney or liver exchange because two donors are required for each recipient. The principle is attractive, however, and the idea that paired exchanges might be managed by a third party (such as United Networks for Organ Sharing) seems worth pursuing.

On several occasions, a living donor has approached the USC transplant program with no relationship of any kind with a potential lung recipient. Given the magnitude of the surgery required for pulmonary lobectomy, USC has been extremely cautious in considering such "good Samaritan" donors, although from a purely ethical point of view they should not be categorically eliminated. Particular attention must be given to the psychosocial evaluation because in some instances "good Samaritans" contacting the authors' team have already donated another organ (ie, kidney) placing them at increased risk for a major procedure.

Commercialism

The issue of allowing commerce to increase the availability of organs for transplant has been exhaustively debated by physicians, economists, and bioethicists. Although in Western countries there remains a consensus that organs should not be subjected to market forces for ethical reasons, other parts of the world take a different view. In Iran thousands of kidney transplants have been performed through a government-sanctioned commercial system of organ distribution. The program has apparently been beneficial to a great number of recipients who otherwise would not have received a transplant [14]. Both sides of the issue need to be looked at carefully.

Those arguing in favor of some form of commerce for transplant organs begin with the right of an individual to be autonomous. The freedom of self-determination should not be stopped because someone chooses to sell a part of oneself. There is also the utilitarian argument that because the volunteer altruistic system is not providing a sufficient number of organs, and because patients can be shown to derive a great benefit from transplant, then an overall good would come from a commercial system that provided more organs. The benefits might outweigh ethical concerns about a reasonable controlled market system [15].

Gill and Sade [16] have presented a provocative argument for why living donors should be allowed to receive payment for a kidney through a tightly regulated agency system that manages acquisition and distribution in a fair and nonexploitive manner. They point out that this does not mean it should be legal for someone to buy an organ. Their case is made in three parts beginning with prima facie argument that a precedent has been established through blood banking that it is ethically and legally acceptable to sell parts of ourselves. Further, individuals have been allowed to donate organs like kidney, liver, and lung; it seems inconsistent to oppose the selling of an organ because of the possible risks, whereas at the same time endorsing donation, which has the same dangers. The authors next challenge arguments that use the Kantian view that selling an organ is intrinsically wrong because it violates the duty of respect for humanity (second formulation of Kant's Categorical Imperative). They point out that selling an organ does not compromise what Kant says is intrinsically valuable, which is the ability to make rational decisions. There is not evidence that giving up a nonvital organ limits future decision making. Finally, Gill and Sade [16] suggest that the potential for exploitation as a result of allowing payment to donors must be evaluated in the context of the loss of lives that could potentially be saved by increasing the number of organs for transplant.

It has also been pointed out that, particularly in the case of end-stage renal disease, transplant provides a significant economic benefit to society [17]. A system to increase the number of transplantable organs may be justified, even if it involves a controlled market.

Do the ends as represented by more organs justify the means, which in this case is commercial vending of human body parts? Kahn and Delmonico [18] succinctly offer arguments against commerce in living donors' organs. These include the basic aversion to the idea of human organs as a commodity; concerns about exploitation; and the risk that commercial donors might withhold important information, such as an underlying illness or transmissible disease, which could cause serious and unmanageable consequences to a potential recipient.

Bioethicists opposed to commercialism of transplantable organs have repeatedly pointed to the risk of exploitations of the poor in favor of the more wealthy in society. Some [19] have attempted, however, to defend organ vending as a way for the less fortunate to lift themselves out of poverty. By pointing out that society has ignored the poor they have argued that one should not stand in the way of a means the poor might have of helping themselves. These arguments, however, represent the minority opinion. Most see commercialism as undermining the moral obligation of society to help the poor, and not leave them in a situation where they must consider selling an organ. Furthermore, it is disturbing that much of the evidence about individuals that have sold an organ suggests that for complex medical, social, economic, and psychosocial reasons, they are worse off after their donation [20].

In a powerful essay on the global traffic in human organs, medical anthropologist Scheper-Hughes [21] has provided a chilling account of what happens to many of those who chose to sell a kidney. Realizing that most donors were from less developed countries (India, Iran, Eastern Europe [particularly Moldova], and the Philippines), postdonation problems including chronic pain, poor overall health, unemployment, reduced income, depression and a sense of worthlessness, family discord, and social isolation were not infrequent. Researchers from Organ Watch (headed by Scheper-Hughes) reported from Iran in regards to major problems with exploitation of the poor despite an attempt by the government to regulate the sale of donor organs. Payment for an organ has been described as "a pittance" and subsequently the seller is said frequently to feel resentment, shame, and family stigma. Anger, resentment, and hostility are also directed at the physicians involved in the harvesting process, which is ethically unacceptable.

Physicians who allow themselves to become involved in organ commerce are subject to serious questioning about their moral values. As described by Delmonico and Surman [22], when patients are marketing their organs, the involved physicians are forced to deal with the dominant financial desires of the would-be-vendor rather than what is medically in the best interest of a patient.

At the worst end of the spectrum are the anecdotal reports of abduction and taking of organs from individuals unable to protect themselves, including in some instances children. Although one would like to think that this never occurs, the possibility remains disturbing.

Although commerce in transplantable organs has been rejected by Western countries, methods legitimately to compensate living donors have been put forward and seem to be gaining acceptance in the transplant community [9,23]. The basic idea is that living donors should not have to bear any costs associated with their act of altruism. Some of the costs are easily reconcilable, such as travel, lodging, and the expenses for testing and hospitalization related to the organ donation. Providing compensation for postoperative outpatient care including such services as physical therapy and long-term follow-up visits also does not seem controversial. Payment for wages lost during medical leave for the donation procedure has been advocated by organizations including the American Society of Transplantation, the Department of Health and Human Services, the Association of Organ Procurement Organizations, and United Networks for Organ Sharing and seems ethically appropriate [24]. It also seems reasonable and morally justifiable to provide financial compensation for insurance against death or disability resulting from the donation procedure. As an extension of this concept, living donors should not lose the ability to obtain health, disability, or life insurance. Compensation to offset additional costs to maintain these programs should not be considered as payment for an organ.

Carrying the concept of compensation further, it has been suggested that incentives in addition to reimbursements might be offered to living donors, although this is clearly crossing into a gray area [25]. Compensation could be given for the pain and suffering in much the same way the legal system allows for such rewards. This type of payment could be considered as a countermeasure to the disincentives of going through a major surgical procedure.

Summary

A constant awareness of the risk to the living donors must be maintained with any living donor organ transplantation program, and comprehensive short- and long-term follow-up should be strongly encouraged to maintain the viability of these potentially life-saving procedures. There has been no perioperative or long-term mortality following lobectomy for living lobar lung transplantation, and perioperative risks associated with donor lobectomy seem to be similar to those seen with standard lung resections [3]. These risks might increase, however, if the procedure is offered on an occasional basis and not within a well-established program.

The long-term outcomes and functional effects of lobar donation raise important questions that are unanswered. This has proved difficult to follow closely, because of the fact that many donors live far from the transplant medical center and are reluctant to return for routine follow-up evaluation. The death of a recipient can further exacerbate this situation, because there is reluctance to insist on further routine examinations for a grieving donor. Prospective donors must be informed of the morbidity associated with lobectomy and the potential for mortality, and for potential negative recipient outcomes in regard to life expectancy and quality of life after transplantation.

Although cadaveric transplantation must be considered because of the risk to the donors, living lobar lung transplantation should continue to be used under properly selected circumstances. The results reported by the authors' group and others [26] are important if this procedure is to be considered as an option at more pulmonary transplant centers in view of the institutional, regional, and international differences in the philosophic and ethical acceptance of the use of living organ donors for transplantation [27].

The integration of ethical discussion into topics that are relevant and of interest to thoracic surgeons, such as living lung donation, is a recent and welcome event. Many of the clinical situations that thoracic surgeons deal with on a daily basis have important and complex ethical implications, and there has been little training to deal effectively with these issues. This is changing as invited discussions on ethically compelling topics are finding their way into journals and the programs of national meetings. What may be of more importance, however, is the development of an ethics curriculum for those training in the specialty. The core curriculum recommended by the Thoracic Surgical Directors Association (which represents the leadership of the 89 approved residency training programs in the United States) has one lecture [28] pertaining to ethics out of the several hundred offerings in its requisite curriculum. It is hoped that this will change in the near future.

References

[1] Moore FD. New problems for surgery. Science 1964; 144:388–92.
[2] Bahaf Arana RJ, Anderson RC, Meyers BF, et al.

Preoperative complications after living donor lobectomy. J Thorac Cardiovasc Surg 2000;120:909–15.
[3] Bowdish ME, Barr ML, Schenkel FA, et al. A decade of living lobar transplantation: perioperative complication after 253 donor lobectomies. Am J Transplant 2004;4:1283.
[4] Beauchamp TL, Childress JF. Principles of biomedical ethics. 5th edition. New York: Oxford University Press; 2001.
[5] Childress JF. Who should decide? Paternalism in health care. New York: Oxford University Press; 1982.
[6] United Networks for Organ Sharing Ethics Committee. Ethics of organ transplantation from living donors. Transplant Proc 1991;24:2236–7.
[7] Woo MS, MacLaughlin EF, Horn MV, et al. Bronchiolitis obliterans is not the primary cause of death in pediatric living donor lobar lung transplant recipients. J Heart Lung Transplant 2001;20:491.
[8] Darr AS, Land W, Yshya TM, et al. Living donor renal transplant: evidence based justification for an ethical option. Transplant Rev 1997;11:95–109.
[9] Abecassis M, Adams M, Adams P, et al. Consensus statement on the live organ donor. JAMA 2000;284: 2919–26.
[10] Barr ML, Bourqu RC, Orens JB, et al. Thoracic organ transplantation in the United States, 1994– 2003. Am J Transplant 2005;5:934–49.
[11] Delmonico FL. Commentary: the WHO resolution on human organ and tissue transplantation. Transplantation 2005;79:639–40.
[12] Terasaki PI, Cecka JM, Giertson DW, et al. High survival rates of kidney transplants from spousal and living unrelated donors. N Engl J Med 1995;333:333–6.
[13] Delmonico FL. Exchanging kidney: advances in living donor transplantation. N Engl J Med 2004; 350:1812.
[14] Ghods AJ. Renal transplantation in Iran. Nephrol Dial Transplant 2002;17:222.
[15] Dosseter J, Levine D. Kidney vending: yes or no? Am J Kidney Dis 2000;35:1002–18.
[16] Gill M, Sade RM. Payment for kidneys: the case for repealing prohibition. Kennedy Inst Ethics J 2002;12: 17–45.
[17] Schnitzler M, Matas A. Paying for living donor (vendor) kidneys: a cost effective analysis. Am J Transplant 2004;4:216–21.
[18] Kahn JP, Delmonico FL. The consequences of public policy to buy and sell organs for transplantation. Am J Transplant 2004;4:178–80.
[19] Radcliffe-Richards J, Darr J, Guttman R, et al. The case for allowing kidney sales. Lancet 1998;351: 1950–2.
[20] Goyal M, Mehta R, Schnederman LJ, et al. Economic and health consequences of selling a kidney in India. JAMA 2002;288:1589–93.
[21] Scheper-Hughes N. Keeping an eye on the global traffic in human organs. Lancet 2003;361:1645–8.
[22] Delmonico FL, Surman O. Is this living donor your patient? Transplantation 2003;76:1257–60.
[23] Delmonico FL, Arnold R, Scheper-Hughes N, et al. Ethical incentives: not payments for organ donation. N Engl J Med 2002;346:2002–5.
[24] American Society of Transplantation. Available at: http://www.a-s-t.org/publicpolicy/organdonation.htm.
[25] Darr AS. Rewarded gifting. Transplant Proc 1992; 24:2207–11.
[26] Date H, Ave M, Sano Y, et al. Improved survival after living-donor lung transplantation. J Thoracic Cardiovasc Surg 2004;128:933.
[27] Patterson GA. Living lobar lung transplantation: is it a necessary option? Am J Transplant 2004;4:1213.
[28] Lytle BW. The ethics of surgical innovation: incorporating emerging technology into surgical practice. TSDA core curriculum 2003. Bethesda (MD): Thoracic Surgery Directors Association; 2003.

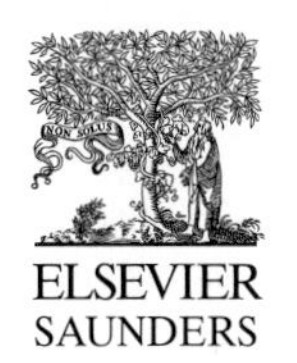

ELSEVIER
SAUNDERS

Thorac Surg Clin 15 (2005) 527 – 532

THORACIC
SURGERY
CLINICS

Conflicts in the Surgeon's Duties to the Patient and Society

Neil J. Farber, MD[a,b,*]

[a]General Internal Medicine Faculty, Christiana Care Health System, 501 West 14th Street, Wilmington, DE 19899, USA
[b]Department of Medicine, Thomas Jefferson University, 111 South 11th Street, Philadelphia, PA 19107, USA

Surgeons often encounter ethical dilemmas in their everyday practice. For example, a frequent issue that surgeons must deal with is whether to initiate or to withdraw life-sustaining treatment [1] and mechanical ventilation [2] in patients who possess or lack decision-making capacity. When facing these dilemmas, surgeons generally weigh competing values, such as the autonomy and rights of the patient, versus beneficence (the best interests of the patient) and nonmaleficence, or avoiding harm [3]. Most of these dilemmas involve only one individual: the patient.

Surgeons may also encounter situations, however, where the competing values involve more than the individual that the surgeon has as a patient. In these cases, the surgeon must weigh the values of autonomy, beneficence, and nonmaleficence on the part of the patient, versus the mandate that society has made along with the beneficence and nonmaleficence toward others. Such issues as deception, confidentiality, and clinical research may pose ethical dilemmas that are sometimes difficult to resolve. This article explores these issues, and provides both guidelines and a mechanism for examining the competing values so that the surgeon can make a decision when faced with these dilemmas. One area that also involves competing values is that of distributive justice [3] (ie, who should receive particular types and amounts of medical care when resources are scarce) [4]. Examples of these dilemmas include who should receive donor hearts [5] and the placement of critically ill patients in ICUs when beds are in short supply [6]. These issues are addressed elsewhere in this issue.

Deception and dishonesty

One of the issues that surgeons may have to deal with is that of honesty and the possibility of deception. It has been stated that it is unethical intentionally to mislead others with deception or outright lies, because society requires truthfulness for individuals to make fully informed choices [7]. The moral duty to refrain from deception also stems from the inherent difficulties with trust that occur if and when an incidence of deception or lying is discovered [8].

Despite the fact that deception and dishonesty are contrary to accepted societal values, some elements of deception and dishonesty have been addressed in the literature. One aspect that has been investigated is the deception and dishonesty that occur during medical training. Such dishonesty might be seen to benefit no one, for the societal view of the profession as a whole may be damaged, and the individual who is dishonest may gain only temporary benefit. Despite this fact, dishonesty and cheating do occur. For example, in one study of second-year medical students [9], 39% of respondents had actually witnessed some type of cheating during the first 2 years of medical school, whereas two thirds reported having heard about such cheating. Deception and dishonesty have also been shown among internal medicine residents [10]. Although residents generally did not deceive their superiors, and especially when the care and medical care of the patient was at stake, over one

The original title was modified to this version by the request of the Guest Editor, Dr. Sade.

* General Internal Medicine Faculty, Christiana Care Health System, 501 West 14th Street, Wilmington, DE 19899.
E-mail address: nfarber@christianacare.org

1547-4127/05/$ – see front matter
doi:10.1016/j.thorsurg.2005.06.011

third of the residents were likely to deceive a fellow resident to avoid switching call. Despite the ethical mandate to avoid deception and dishonesty, among medical students and residents it is practiced when care of the patient is not an issue.

Dishonesty and deception can also at times involve the patient. The question of whether to inform patients about bad news, such as cancer, is no longer an issue for surgeons. In one study [11], 98% of physicians who were surveyed in one academic institution indicated that their policy was generally to tell their patients about the diagnosis of cancer. Only 25 years previously, however, 69% of physicians indicated that they generally did not or never told their patients about such a diagnosis [12]. This change in attitude toward the information patients have the right to know is caused by a rise in consumerism and a parallel decline in paternalism on the part of the physician [11].

A more recent conflict in communication with patients involves the disclosure of medical errors. In deciding whether to disclose a medical error to a patient, physicians must weigh patient autonomy (the right of a patient to know the information) versus the potential financial and social harm to the physician [13]. In addition, the potential for societal harm exists if information is withheld from patients, because there may be a decline in public confidence in physicians. It has been stated that because of the precedence of patient autonomy, physicians have an ethical obligation to disclose all medical errors to patients [14,15]. Most physicians are in agreement with the need to disclose such errors to patients. In one study [5], 95% of respondent physicians indicated they would disclose a medical error that resulted in a prolonged hospitalization with consequent back pain, and 84% indicated that they would disclose an error that resulted in the death of a patient. In another survey [16], over one half of respondents would inform a family of a medication error that led to the death of a patient. Surgeons also have a practical reason for disclosing medical errors to patients: patients who have sued physicians indicated that dishonesty about a medical error was a major reason for their decision to sue [17].

Another way in which dishonesty or deception may play a role in the care of patients is that of the use of placebos. Placebos have been accepted for their use in research involving controlled drug trials. Prescribing placebos to one's patients in a clinical practice has been believed to be unethical, however, because of the deception that is involved [18]. This deception is believed to be an abuse of power on the part of the physician that deprives the patient of both dignity and autonomy [19], not withstanding the beneficence that may occur. Deception may also be harmful to the society, because of the mistrust that may occur and the loss of respect for physicians by other health care workers [20]. Despite these ethical concerns 28% of internal medicine residents and subspecialty fellows had given a placebo to patients outside of a clinical trial [21].

One way in which placebos can be given to patients outside of a clinical trial is if the surgeon uses no deception or dishonesty in its use. One author [22] has advocated the introduction of a written agreement in which the patient is informed that at some point in the patient's care a placebo may be introduced. Such an agreement, however, still entails an element of deception in that the placebo is not identified as such. It has been noted that placebos have limited clinical applicability as long as deception and dishonesty are avoided [23]. The best guideline to follow in regards to placebos is to avoid their use and thereby avoid the deception that is likely to accompany them.

Some surgeons may believe that deception may be acceptable as long as it is in the best interest of the patient. Such a situation may occur when a surgeon believes it is necessary to falsify information to have a patient obtain care (eg, a radiologic procedure) that otherwise is not covered by his or her medical insurance. This situation clearly pits the best interest (beneficence) of a patient versus the beneficence or nonmaleficence of the society as a whole. Many physicians are concerned about the lack of coverage by medical insurers of routine screening and preventative care [24]. Patients could get care that is otherwise denied to them (and for which they may not have the financial reserves to pay) if the surgeon is willing to fudge or manipulate the medical information of the patient. Conversely, at least financial harm may occur to society when such actions are taken by surgeons, In addition, as with any type of dishonesty, patient trust in the physician might be eroded. In more serious cases, other patients may be denied medical services that they require, for example in the case of a patient who is cared for in the surgical ICU when they do not meet the criteria necessary for a surgical ICU stay.

Studies have shown that some physicians are likely to "game the system" to have medical insurers pay for medical care they believe is in the best interest of the patient. Thirty-nine percent of practicing physicians who were surveyed in one study [25] indicated that they had at least sometimes or often used one or more of three tactics for manipulating reimbursement rules. These tactics included exaggerating the severity of a patient's symptoms, changing a patient's billing diagnosis, and recording signs or symptoms that the patient actually did not have. In another study [16], almost 70% of physicians were willing to give a diagnosis of "rule out cancer" to have a mammogram paid for by a third-party payor. Although some [24] have argued against the use of deception to achieve a manipulation of the reimbursement system, the surgeon who is faced with this dilemma must carefully weigh his or her obligation to the individual patient versus the obligations to the society as a whole.

Confidentiality

No issue highlights the conflicts surgeons may face in dealing with the rights of an individual versus those of society [26] more than that of confidentiality. This conflict occurs because surgeons have a fiduciary responsibility to an individual that is based on trust [27], with this responsibility requiring the protection of that individual's rights and autonomy. The surgeon also, however, has an obligation to others' interests, especially when societal harm may ensue from fulfilling the responsibility to one individual. For example, patients with various diseases have the right to have the information that they have their illness kept confidential; however, when that disease is communicable, it presents a danger to specific others who have contacted that individual, and in some cases, to the society as a whole. Surgeons have a legal requirement to report such cases to the public health department [28].

A more difficult decision, however, is whether to inform a sexual partner of an individual who is infected with a sexually transmitted disease. Reporting of such an individual to the public health department, as is required, is unlikely to protect the sexual partner from the potential of contracting that sexually transmitted disease. The surgeon must decide whether still to maintain the patient's confidentiality, or whether to breach that confidentiality to protect the sexual partner. There is a great deal of controversy about whether confidentiality should be breached in such cases. One area of greatest controversy exists in the decision to breach confidentiality to a sexual partner of a patient infected with HIV [29]. Several societies, such as the American Medical Association (AMA) and the American College of Emergency Physicians, have indicated that physicians should inform the sexual partner of an HIV-infected patient, but only when the patient refuses to inform the partner [30]. No statutes exist on the subject [25], and case law has ruled both for and against maintaining confidentiality even in cases of impending harm to another individual [30]. When faced with a similar situation, a surgeon must weigh the competing ethical values in making his or her decision.

Another aspect of the risk to society involves individuals who are impaired in some fashion. One particular concern is the automobile driver with seizures. Although only six states actually require physicians to report patients who have epilepsy, case law has indicated that physicians have an obligation to breach confidentiality and report impaired drivers in these cases [31]. In situations where the society is at significant risk from an impaired individual (eg, automobile, bus, and tractor-trailer drivers and pilots) because of any cause (eg, seizures, alcohol intoxication, or syncopal episodes), the surgeon does have an obligation to breach confidentiality and inform the appropriate authorities. A more troubling situation for many physicians is the impaired colleague. The AMA's Code of Medical Ethics clearly states that physicians do have an obligation to report any impaired colleagues [32]. Physicians may fail to report an impaired colleague, however, so as to protect the colleague from adverse social, financial, and legal consequences [33]. In addition, the social stigmatization of both the impaired physician and the accusing physician may be preventing them from doing so. Although 65% of physicians have indicated that they would report an impaired colleague because of alcohol, drugs, or a mental or physical ailment [34], physicians more often would report colleagues impaired because of substance abuse than those cognitively or psychologically impaired [35]. Surgeons need to be informed about the availability of Physicians' Health Programs and the ethical obligation of reporting their impaired colleagues.

Some thoracic surgeons may occasionally encounter a situation in which a patient requires surgery because of a gunshot or stab wound. In these situations, most states have laws that mandate the reporting of such criminally inflicted injuries to the police and other authorities [30]. In situations where a patient indicates that he or she plans violent action against another specified individual, precedents such as the Tarasoff decision [36] indicate that the surgeon has a duty to warn both the authorities and the intended victim [37]. In balancing the right of privacy of the patient with the nonmaleficence of another individual, the surgeon has an obligation to breach confidentiality. In addition to liability for the failure to warn an intended victim, however, surgeons may be exposed to liability if they release information where there is no clear danger or specified victim

[38]. Despite the need for future, intended harm to a specific individual before a physician should breach confidentiality, it has been found that residents in internal medicine were likely to breach confidentiality even when such elements were absent in hypothetical cases [39]. Surgeons should consult their state laws and case decisions when deciding to breach confidentiality when a clear danger exists for another individual.

Although it is clear that surgeons may not participate in patients' attempts at engaging in health insurance fraud [40], occasionally a patient may disclose the fact that they had engaged in such behaviors in the past. The surgeon may then be faced with the ethical dilemma of protecting the privacy of the patient, versus the financial harm that may come to society. Most states do not require physicians to disclose insurance fraud [41]. From an ethical point of view, however, it has been noted that surgeons should maintain confidentiality of patients' information unless there is a threat of bodily harm to another individual, laws that require reporting, or a need to protect another individual or societal interest [42]. Patients expect that such sensitive information would be withheld from insurance companies [43], yet most physicians who were surveyed indicated that they would report past occurrence of patient-initiated insurance fraud under certain circumstances [44]. In cases where patients reveal past occurrences of insurance fraud, surgeons must weigh the obligation they have to maintain patient confidentiality versus the society's interest in preventing and recouping financial losses.

Clinical research

Medical research creates a risk for an individual patient that may in consequence benefit future individuals. It has been said that this conflict between serving the needs of an individual patient and benefiting humankind with new knowledge is often a difficult dilemma [45] for society, and it certainly is no less so for the clinician-researcher.

Surgeons often are called on by patients to give advice concerning clinical trials, and often refer such patients to investigators for enrollment into studies. Some surgeons also conduct or participate in research studies using human subjects, whereas others may sit on institutional review boards, which are responsible for review of the various research protocols. This topic is addressed elsewhere in this issue in the article by Miller.

Acting as an agent of society

In some situations, a surgeon may be asked to use his or her medical skills as a mandate from the society, rather than as a physician caring for a patient. One prototypic example of this occurrence is involvement in the process of lethal injection for the purposes of capital punishment. Legal and societal imperatives exist that require physicians actively to participate in the process of lethal injection for the purpose of capital punishment. For example, 27 states require or permit physicians to be involved in the process of capital punishment [46]. At the same time, there is an ethical imperative within the medical profession for physicians to avoid participating in lethal injections. The Council on Ethical and Judicial Affairs of the American Medical Association [47] has published guidelines that state that it is unethical for physicians to engage in most aspects of lethal injection. There is also a consensus in the ethics literature that physicians should not participate in lethal injections, because participation violates the principle of nonmaleficence [48].

Physicians' attitudes about involvement in capital punishment may be dependent on a number of factors that individuals must weigh. One of these factors might involve a comparison of one's responsibility to the individual versus the duty to society [49]. Pellegrino [50] has pointed out that in cases involving capital punishment, physicians face competing values: the requirement to fulfill legally or socially prescribed roles as an agent of the society as a whole, versus a responsibility to the patient as a member of the medical profession. It has been found that most physicians condone colleagues' involvement in at least some aspects of the lethal injection process [51], and some physicians were willing actually to participate in capital punishment in association with their perceived duty to society [52]. Given the consensus by the AMA and most ethicists that it is unethical for physicians to participate in executions, any surgeon who is asked to participate in the lethal injection process must carefully examine their obligation to do no harm to others. In a similar manner, it has been suggested that physicians should not participate in the interrogation of prisoners [53].

Summary

Surgeons may face a dilemma in which their obligations to their patients and their obligations to others or society may conflict. One way of examining these conflicts is through a model as depicted in Fig. 1.

		Individual	
		Benefit	Burden
Society	Benefit	Positive effects for both--can proceed	Conflict--those who support the Rights of society
	Burden	Conflict--those who support the rights of an individual	Negative effects for both--should avoid

Fig. 1. Assessing conflicts between individuals and society.

When both the patient and society are benefited (eg, in cases of routine surgical care), the surgeon may proceed with the planned treatment. In situations where it is agreed that both the patient and society will be harmed (eg, surgeon involvement in capital punishment or in many cases of deception), the surgeon should avoid acting in a manner against that of the patient. Many situations, however, involve the need to weigh the benefits and burdens of both the patient and society. In these cases, surgeons need to analyze carefully all of the ethical and legal issues involved, and make a decision based on their own set of values.

References

[1] Ruark JE, Raffin TA. The Stanford University Medical Center Committee on Ethics Initiating and withdrawing life support: principles and practice in adult medicine. N Engl J Med 1988;318:25–30.

[2] Schneiderman LJ, Spragg RGN. Ethical decisions in discontinuing mechanical ventilation. N Engl J Med 1988;318:984–8.

[3] Young EWD. Ethical issues in medicine. In: Alpha & omega: ethics at the frontiers of life and death. Menlo Park (CA): Addison-Wesley; 1989. p. 14–26.

[4] Sprung CL, Eidelman LA, Steinberg A. Is the physician's duty to the individual patient or to society? Crit Care Med 1995;23:618–9.

[5] Dracup K. Saying no and other ethical dilemmas. Heart Lung 1986;15:1–2.

[6] Engelhardt HT, Rie MA. Intensive care units, scarce resources, and conflicting principles of justice. JAMA 1986;255:1159–64.

[7] Young TA. Teaching medical students to lie. The disturbing contradiction: medical ideals and the resident-selection process. Can Med Assoc J 1997;156:219–22.

[8] Gillon R. Is there an important moral distinction for medical ethics between lying and other forms of deception? J Med Ethics 1993;19:131–2.

[9] Baldwin Jr DC, Daugherty SR, Rowley BD, et al. Cheating in medical school: a survey of second-year students at 31 schools. Acad Med 1996;71:267–73.

[10] Green MJ, Farber NJ, Ubel PA, et al. Lying to each other: when internal medicine residents use deception with their colleagues. Arch Intern Med 2000;160: 2317–23.

[11] Novack DH, Plumer R, Smith RL, et al. Changes in physicians' attitudes toward telling the cancer patient. JAMA 1979;241:897–900.

[12] Fitt Jr WT, Ravdin IS. What Philadelphia physicians tell patients with cancer. JAMA 1953;153: 901–4.

[13] Wu AW, Cavanaugh TA, McPhee SJ, et al. To tell the truth: ethical and practical issues in disclosing medical mistakes to patients. J Gen Intern Med 1997;12: 770–7.

[14] Rosner F, Berger JT, Kark P, et al. Disclosure and prevention of medical errors. Arch Intern Med 2000; 160:2089–92.

[15] Sweet MP, Bernat JL. A study of the ethical duty of physicians to disclose errors. J Clin Ethics 1997;8: 341–8.

[16] Novack DH, Detering BJ, Arnold R, et al. Physicians' attitudes toward using deception to resolve difficult ethical problems. JAMA 1989;261:2980–5.

[17] Vincent C, Young M, Phillips A. Why do people sue doctors? A study of patients and relatives taking legal action. Lancet 1994;343:1609–13.

[18] Markus AC. The ethics of placebo prescribing. Mt Sinai J Med 2000;67:140–3.

[19] Bakhurst D. On lying and deceiving. J Med Ethics 1992;18:63–6.

[20] Hill J. Placebos in clinical care: for whose pleasure? Lancet 2003;362:254.

[21] Green MJ, Mitchell G, Stocking CB, et al. Do actions reported by physicians in training conflict with consensus guidelines on ethics? Arch Intern Med 1996; 156:298–304.

[22] Lione A. Ethics of placebo use in clinical care. Lancet 2003;362:999.

[23] Brody H. The lie that heals: the ethics of giving placebos. Ann Intern Med 1982;97:112–8.

[24] Morreim EH. Gaming the system: dodging the rules, ruling the dodgers. Arch Intern Med 1991;151:443–7.

[25] Wynia MK, Cummins DS, VanGeest JB, et al. Physician manipulation of reimbursement rules for patients: between a rock and a hard place. JAMA 2000;283:1858–65.

[26] Melroe NH. Duty to warn vs. patient confidentiality: the ethical dilemmas in caring for HIV-infected clients. Nurse Pract 1990;15:58–69.

[27] Perkins HS, Jonsen AR. Conflicting duties to patients: the case of a sexually active hepatitis B carrier. Ann Intern Med 1981;94(Part 1):523–30.

[28] Report of the Council on Ethical and Judicial Affairs of the American Medical Association. No. 26. Chicago: AMA; 1990.

[29] Huprich SK, Fuller KM, Schneider RB. Divergent ethical perspectives on the duty-to-warn principle with HIV patients. Ethics Behav 2003;13:263–78.

[30] Larkin GL, Moskop J, Sanders A, et al. The emergency

physician and patient confidentiality: a review. Ann Emerg Med 1994;24:1161–7.
[31] Krumholz A, Fisher RS, Lesser RP, et al. Driving and epilepsy: a review and reappraisal. JAMA 1991;265: 622–6.
[32] Goldrich MS. Reporting impaired, incompetent or unethical colleagues, amendment. AMA Council on Ethical and Judicial Affairs, June 2004. Available at: www.ama-assn.org/ama1/pub/upload/mm/369/rprtcolleag_ceja_a04.pdf. Accessed March 7, 2005.
[33] Terry K. Impaired physicians: speak no evil? Med Econ 2002;79:110–7.
[34] McCall SV. Chemically dependent health professionals. West J Med 2001;174:50–4.
[35] Farber NJ, Gilibert S, Aboff BM, et al. Physicians' willingness to report impaired colleagues. Soc Sci Med 2005;61:1772–5.
[36] Quinn KM. The impact of Tarasoff on clinical practice. Behav Sci Law 1984;2:319–29.
[37] Annas GJ. Confidentiality and the duty to warn. Hastings Cent Rep 1976;6:6–8.
[38] Roth LH, Meisel A. Dangerousness, confidentiality, and the duty to warn. Am J Psychiatry 1977;134:508–11.
[39] Farber NJ, Weiner JL, Boyer EG, et al. Residents' decisions to breach confidentiality. J Gen Intern Med 1989;4:31–3.
[40] Khajezadeh D. Patient confidentiality statutes in Medicare and Medicaid fraud investigations. Am J Law Med 1987;13:105–37.
[41] Appelbaum PS, Meisel A. Therapists' obligations to report their patients' criminal acts. Bull Am Acad Psychiatry Law 1986;14:221–30.
[42] Council on Ethical and Judicial Affairs. Fundamental elements of the patient-physician relationship. In: Reports of the Council on Ethical and Judicial Affairs. Chicago: American Medical Association; 1990. p. 1–4.
[43] Lorge RE. How informed is patients' consent to release of medical information to insurance companies? BMJ 1989;298:1495–6.
[44] Farber NJ, Berger MS, Davis EB, et al. Confidentiality and health insurance fraud. Arch Intern Med 1997;157: 501–4.
[45] Annas GJ. Questing for grails: duplicity, betrayal, and self-deception in postmodern medical research. J Contemp Health Law Policy 1996;12:297–323.
[46] Skolnick AA. Physicians in Missouri (but not Illinois) win battle to block physician participation in executions. JAMA 1995;274:524.
[47] Council on Ethical and Judicial Affairs of the American Medical Association. Physician participation in capital punishment. JAMA 1993;270:365–8.
[48] Rosner F, Halpern AL, Kark PR, et al. Physician involvement in capital punishment. N Y State J Med 1991;91:15–8.
[49] Thorburn KM. Physicians and the death penalty. West J Med 1987;146:638–40.
[50] Pellegrino ED. Societal duty and moral complicity: the physician's dilemma of divided loyalty. Int J Law Psychiatry 1993;16:371–91.
[51] Farber NJ, Davis EB, Weiner J, et al. Physicians' attitudes about involvement in lethal injection for capital punishment. Arch Intern Med 2000;160:2912–6.
[52] Farber NJ, Aboff BM, Weiner J, et al. Physicians' willingness to participate in the process of lethal injection for capital punishment. Ann Intern Med 2001; 135:884–8.
[53] Bloche MG, Marks JH. When doctors go to war. N Engl J Med 2005;352:3–6.

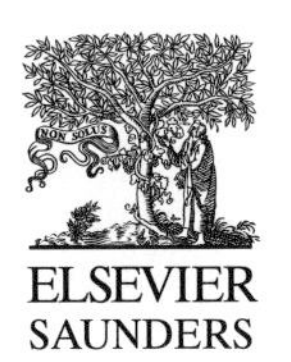

ELSEVIER
SAUNDERS

Thorac Surg Clin 15 (2005) 533 – 542

THORACIC
SURGERY
CLINICS

Who's Buying Lunch: Are Gifts to Surgeons from Industry Bad for Patients?

David C. Grant, MD, ARDMS*, Kenneth V. Iserson, MD, MBA, FACEP

Department of Emergency Medicine, University of Arizona College of Medicine, 1501 North Campbell Avenue, PO Box 24-5057, Tucson, AZ 85724, USA

Although both medicine and business are ethical activities, they are not the same ethical activity [1]

Drug company marketing is focused on physicians and surgeons, because they, rather than their patients, are usually the de facto purchasers. Pharmaceutical advertising is an investment that buys professional trust. The aim is to increase profits, and that occurs if clinicians recognize and identify with their brand. This, however, conflicts with public perceptions and expectations. Patients entrust the medical profession with a fiduciary role in managing and distributing their health care resources, expecting that physicians use their professional knowledge and experience objectively to prescribe medications.

Industry marketing to surgeons

Direct marketing to physicians proliferates despite attempts at regulation. In the United States more than one third of the industry's promotional budget is allotted to detailing, and there is approximately one pharmaceutical sales representative for every 15 physicians [2]. At the start of the 1990s, estimates of United States promotional spending ranged from $2.5 [3] to $5 billion [4], or $5000 per year per physician [5].

Despite recognition of potential harm, the 1990s were a decade of incredible growth in detailing. In 1999, the pharmaceutical industry spent nearly $8 billion to send sales representatives to physician offices and exhibit products at medical conferences and events [6]. By 2001 annual promotion exceeded $11 billion, with $8000 to $13,000 spent directly or indirectly per year on each physician [7]. In 2002, one third of gross revenue went to sales and administration, and Novartis reported (in 2001) spending 36% of revenue on marketing alone [8,9]. By 2003, direct to physician advertising reached $22 billion, and the retail value of sample gifts was a staggering $16 billion [10].

Surgeons are not immune from detailing, being frequent targets of gifts from equipment company representatives and the more widely studied pharmaceutical representatives, referred to as "detail" men and women. Industry representatives are the most beautiful, friendliest, helpful, persistent, flattering group anyone meets. They project the opposite of a zero-sum game, the limits of a health care system in crisis are not mentioned, and everyone should feel good about little rewards for their hard work.

Although surveyed physicians typically deny that gifts influence their medical practice, they concede that they would have less contact with detailers if they received no promotional items (positive reinforcement), and this practice correlates with a belief that gifts produce no impact on prescribing behavior [11].

Industry representatives purchase time with surgeons and physicians using meals (including the lunches served at teaching conferences); toys; pens; books; tickets to sporting events; travel; and medical samples donated to clinics. They use this time, to the

* Corresponding author.
E-mail address: grantdav77@hotmail.com (D.C. Grant).

1547-4127/05/$ – see front matter
doi:10.1016/j.thorsurg.2005.06.004

extent possible, to demonstrate company devices and market new medications or new uses for their current medications. Surgical residencies frequently rely on drug company funding for educational lunches and speaker fees. Medical students receive books, meals, and occasionally travel to surgical conferences, perhaps to acculturate them.

Surgeons, as professionals often under psychologic pressures, are subject to enticements. The surgical literature, however, is almost devoid of ethical commentary on the subject of receiving gifts. There are no published data differentiating surgeons from other physicians. Additionally, device marketers may be more effective than "pill pushers" at getting an audience with surgeons. Mark Bard, president of Manhattan Research LLC (a pharmaceutical marketing firm) commented in an industry journal in 2003 that "Clinical users want to see and feel new devices or products, but they do not need to see or feel pills" [12].

Gifts from drug companies sometimes take the form of free medicine, but the pharmaceutical and medical device industries are not in the business of providing free care. The free samples are provided, of course, to promote the newest, most expensive medications.

Industry defense of detailing

Although there is little in the medical literature defending detailing, the pharmaceutical industry makes the following arguments.

Professionals can and should use judgment

Regulation is an unnecessary imposition on physicians who have dedicated their careers to careful scrutiny of data and patient care. Doctors are trained in ethics, have good characters, and do not abuse their positions; they are not petty. Bert Spilker, a senior vice-president of scientific and regulatory affairs at Pharmaceutical Research and Manufacturers of America (PhRMA) wrote "...(Critics of detailing) fear that physicians are so weak and lacking in integrity that they would 'sell their souls' for a pack of M&M candies and a few sandwiches and doughnuts...certainly the vast majority of physicians are able to resist this temptation and make decisions solely based on the best medical interests of their patients" [13].

This country has a long-standing tradition of allowing professional medical societies and boards to police their own, and many in the United States now enjoy the most technologically advanced system of medical care in the world. Caring for patients, and not self-interest, motivates physicians and their judgment should be trusted.

The research, development, and sale of pharmaceuticals requires physician contact

In the competitive marketplace there is a race to bring new technologies to the patient. Physicians are positioned to participate in trials, author papers, and benefit from efficient notification of advantageous devices and drugs. Gifts and meals are fair reimbursement for time spent interacting with the representative. It is a win-win situation. Patients receive the latest medical care and companies with superior ideas have a platform to present them and evaluate their performance [13]. Furthermore, a firm that does not aggressively market to physicians is at a competitive disadvantage, even if it offers a safer or more efficacious product.

Detailing is standard of care in a free market system

The delivery of health care is best accomplished by allowing profit motive to attract providers to consumers. Just as superior products survive, the lowest cost provision of good care flourishes. If there is any doubt, just look at the failed state-planned health systems of Eastern Europe, and unacceptable delay for elective procedures in Canada and the United Kingdom. Marketing is education. Physicians who decline to associate with detailers should not be allowed to impose on those who benefit from the exchange of ideas. The economy thrives on liberty; detailing is necessary for physician acceptance of new information.

Small gifts do not affect physician behavior

The recently adopted PhRMA code ensures that gifts are insignificant (like M&Ms) and pertain directly to improvement in patient care. Anatomic models, books, and patient information brochures are convenient and meaningful for the physician and patient, but they are not for personal consumption [14]. Although meals for physicians and clinic staff are appreciated, they are too modest to constitute an enticement to change practice patterns.

Drug samples help the poor

Millions of doses of the newest and most effective medications are distributed freely to patients that otherwise could not afford them. Some inner city and rural clinics rely on pharmaceutical samples to provide modern care for their poorest patients. Even insured patients benefit. Gerald Mossinghoff, president of the PhRMA, testified at a hearing before the Senate Committee on Labor and Human Resources in 1990 that samples:

> Allow physicians to initiate therapy immediately in their office, which is important for urgent and painful conditions. In addition the physician can evaluate the effect of the drug, detect any early side effects in the patient, and adjust the prescribed dosage before a full prescription is paid for by the patient. Samples thus provide a convenient mechanism to achieve the best available therapy without forcing the patient to incur costs for a drug that may not work for him or her [15].

Regulation of detailing

Regulations governing pharmaceutical detailing stem from the medical profession (voluntary and very weak); the pharmaceutical industry (voluntary and somewhat stronger); and court-enforced legislation (strong, because they have financial penalties attached). In 1987, the American Surgical Association acknowledged the potent effect of pharmaceutical gifts and resolved "that it is unethical for a surgeon to accept...material reward for participating in...product promotional activity...with no relationship to professional service rendered by the surgeon" [16].

On December 3, 1990, the American Medical Association's (AMA) Council on Ethical and Judicial Affairs issued a largely unpopular opinion concerning gifts to physicians from industry. It said that gifts should primarily benefit the patient and should not be of substantial value. Textbooks, modest meals, and other gifts were appropriate if they serve an educational function. Medical equipment is included in a clarifying addendum to the 1990 opinion; devices cannot be of substantial value, and the relevant measure of their cost is whatever the surgeon needs to pay to purchase the item on the open market [17]. Subsidies to underwrite the costs of continuing medical education are permissible but need to be accepted by the conference's sponsor and not given directly to the physician. No gifts should be accepted if there are strings attached, [18] and gifts...

> ought not to be accepted if acceptance might influence or appear to others to influence the objectivity of clinical judgment. A useful criterion in determining acceptable activities and relationships is: Would you be willing to have these arrangements generally known? [19]

These recommendations were straightforward but nonbinding, and clearly allowed for frequent small gifts and meals.

In 2003, the nation's largest hospital system, the Veteran's Health Administration (VHA), adopted stricter rules of conduct for drug company sales representatives. It specifies that marketing visits must be at the invitation of the Veteran's Administration staff, representatives are not allowed to attend medical conferences, food items must be of nominal value and not include meals, outright gifts cannot exceed $20 per occurrence, and no more than $50 in aggregate value over a consecutive 12-month period from any one source [20]. It is unclear what enforcement mechanisms exist.

One private group, "No Free Lunch" (www.nofreelunch.org), educates and organizes health care providers to reject detailing. Members pledge to accept no money, gifts, or hospitality from the pharmaceutical industry and to avoid conflicts of interest in practice, teaching, or research. This includes pens, coffee mugs, and especially lunch [21]. The only United States professional group to espouse complete detachment of industry from physicians is the American Medical Student Association [22]. This may reflect youthful idealism, or the seeds of a cultural shift.

Beginning in the late 1990s, egregious marketing schemes began to attract judicial challenges based on laws intended for other purposes. In the 1990s, passage of the False Claims Act imposed civil liability, including treble damage awards plus up to $11,000 per claim, on individuals or businesses that knowingly seek to defraud the federal government. The Act bolsters the 1972 antikickback law designed to protect the Medicare and Medicaid programs against fraudulent expenditures [23]. In 1997, a former Takeda Chemical Industries and Abbott Laboratories (TAP pharmaceuticals) employee revealed that TAP employed doctors as "consultants" and took physicians on free trips and awarded educational grants. The physicians did not bill TAP for their time and increases in revenue from TAP's leuprolide acetate, an expensive gonadotropin agonist, were argued by federal prosecutors to have resulted from kickbacks to the physicians. TAP settled with the government for $290 million in criminal fines plus $585 million in civil penalties; the whistle-blowers received nearly $100 million [23].

Based on effective litigation of TAP, in 2003 AstraZeneca settled criminal fraud charges of

$355 million that involved similar inducements to increase drug sales of its own gonadotropin agonist, goserelin acetate [24]. Currently, Schering-Plough faces ongoing investigation for the alleged use of sham consultants with the hepatitis drug interferon alfa-2b [25]. The prosecution of individual physicians in this case exposes doctors to unprecedented types of financial risk.

The pharmaceutical industry responded by adopting its own ethical code. These nonbinding guidelines, unanimously approved on April 18, 2002, by PhRMA, became effective for the 82,000 detail men and women [26] in the United States on July 1, 2002 [14]. The PhRMA code allows industry representatives to provide meals as long as they are "modest." No entertainment or recreational activities are permitted. Items primarily for the benefit of the patient under $100 are acceptable [14]. The effect of letting the foxes guard the henhouse has not become apparent, but by formally sanctioning gifts under $100 per visit, industry provides a solid target to debate ethically. One bright spot springs from the Office of the Inspector General of the Department of Health and Human Services, which requires the pharmaceutical companies to comply with the new PhRMA Code [27]. But the Office of the Inspector General also admonishes that the drug companies "separate their grant-making functions from their sales and marketing functions" [28]. The contention that education and promotion can be mutually exclusive is probably wrong.

Even with Code compliance, the problem is not solved by high-profile court settlements. The bulk of gifts to surgeons are difficult to find and individually inconsequential. Their reach is cumulative and insidious. Effecting behavioral change in a competitive marketplace requires enforcement and detection mechanisms, and a shift in physician ethics.

Gift theory

> Equo ne credite, Teucri. Quidquid id est, timeo Danaos et dona ferentis (Do not trust the horse, Trojans. Whatever it is, I fear the Greeks even when they bring gifts). Virgil 70–19 BC

The acceptance of a gift forms a relationship whereby the recipient is indebted to the giver. The timing and magnitude of gifting is culturally directed. There is little randomness. In certain situations gifts of a specific value are expected. Why does the custom continue despite the simplicity of financial transactions in modern society? The answer is relationships. The bond between recipient and gift giver is impossible to measure, but very real. Traditionally, strangers do not give one another gifts unless an exchange of favors is expected.

A gift is something given, not purchased. Virtually any resource can be transformed into a gift. This applies to tangibles and intangible assistance [29]. In primitive societies, gifts form the basis for relationships, with members working toward common goals that unite them and create the expectation of future assistance in time of need. Adroit individuals probably exploited the exchange to gain control. This behavior eventually became institutionalized and a part of every culture [30]. Only the most aberrant social behavior lacks an element of exchange [29].

What is a bribe? The simplest answer is a gift with strings attached, although the boundary is indistinct and must be defined on a cultural basis [31]. Social scientists agree that the prevailing purpose of gifts is to establish the identity of the donor and encourage reciprocity [32]. Gifts that seem inappropriately generous are bribes. Although inexpensive gifts foster relationships, the acceptance of bribes might imply prepayment for some future action that benefits the giver. Both gifts and bribes create reciprocity, but bribes are a step closer to specifying the magnitude of compensation. A risk to the surgeon accepting some gifts is that they may meet the definition (in spirit, if not in law) of bribes.

In the business world gifts create a tension that is relieved by repayment. The implicit recognition of dependence on the giver burdens the recipient with a loss of status and self-esteem if there is a failure to repay [30]. The "reactance" theory argues that the degree of expected reciprocity correlates with a loss of freedom. Individuals, or companies, have the opportunity to shed this encumbrance with repayment. Perhaps the most ironic example of corporate resistance of employee gifts is the pharmaceutical industry itself. Merck, Upjohn, Eli Lilly, and Abbott Laboratories all have policies that either forbid the acceptance of gifts or limit their value to $5 or $10. The purchasing manager at Eli Lilly and Company, Indianapolis, Indiana, commented, "We want to keep things straight, aboveboard, business" [33]. He is aware that accepting a gift predicts future favoritism toward the giver, and the response may take an unprofitable course from the company's perspective.

It is also instructive to see who does not give physicians gifts. Although they are the only large profession in the highest 10% of United States income, physicians do not receive gifts from those who wish to solicit their personal business, such as automobile lots or jewelry stores. When, for example, was the last time Mercedes-Benz or Microsoft advertised in general medical journals? Physicians receive gifts when they spend other peoples' money, not their own.

Drug companies understand that even inexpensive tokens generate reciprocity. Although large items might engender greater appreciation from clinicians, they raise the question of impropriety and risk third-party criticism. Worse still, extravagant offerings might be declined, and the strain could sever an otherwise productive relationship. Small items are ideal. They are inconspicuous. The public seldom knows or cares. For example, a survey of family practice patients in Missouri revealed only 17.5% disapproves of physicians accepting pens from detailers [34]. As many physician recipients say: even if a pen displays a proprietary logo it is still just a pen. Furthermore, PhRMA, AMA, and VHA condone these gifts.

The three types of more expensive direct gifts to physicians that survived current PhRMA and AMA guidelines are meals, medication and equipment samples, and educational items. Each of these gift types is engineered to establish a relationship with the physician. Mealtime is social and pleasant. People generally stop working and share something of themselves. The gift of time, food, friendship, and flattery cements personal relationships [8] that industry blurs into business commitments. Even lunchtime lectures allow for 10 minutes of small talk beforehand. The representative is a provider of good feelings and closeness, both of which engender trust. Many physicians are not seasoned business-types and probably are unaware of this subtle, but effective, marketing [35].

There is another important permissive factor: patient ignorance. There is very little accountability in the business of medicine. Patients pay for the gifts through higher drug and equipment (built into higher hospital costs) prices, but rarely know that their physician even accepts gifts [36]. In economic theory the costs they bear are externalities. An externality is something that does not factor into the immediate transaction, although it affects the transaction. When surgeons neglect to inform their patients that they dine with drug or equipment company representatives, the true cost of their indulgence is hidden. The ultimate consumers who must pay the bill, the patients, are omitted from the transaction.

Samples

Industry defends samples in terms of humanitarian aid and patient convenience. Many physicians appreciate samples and the AMA even approves personal use of drug samples for practicing doctors and their families as long as these practices do not interfere with patient access to samples [23]. Enforcement of this "interference" is not practical; when the cupboard is bare the representatives probably just bring more samples.

Sample medications are, overall, the most expensive gifts given to physicians (individual trips, medical equipment, grants, and consulting fees are more expensive, but are much less commonly dispersed). This is because of the high retail prices for the new drugs distributed as samples. They are given with the expectation that the patients often stay on them for an entire course, and sometimes chronically, and that the physician becomes comfortable using the drug in place of alternatives. Sample medications and educational items, such as books, may exceed "small" gift categorization without attracting too much criticism because the perception that there is a direct patient benefit seems to mitigate any impropriety.

Samples are also an effective marketing device. Samples are never generic, and seldom for inexpensive therapy. They lower the bar for beginning, or fostering the habit of prescribing, an expensive new therapy. Accepting samples was associated with awareness, preference, and rapid prescription of a new drug [37]. In a survey of family practice residents, 55% admitted that samples biased their prescribing [38].

Irrational prescribing notwithstanding, sample diversion is a serious issue. Samples are sometimes resold, stolen, or appropriated by office staff. An observational study of family practitioner office use of samples in New York state discovered that approximately one third of the medications were diverted to physicians and their families or had an unknown destination [39].

There is a paucity of education associated with dispensed samples. Direct observation of 1588 family practice visits in Nebraska in 1999 revealed that less than one half of samples dispensed included even verbal instructions, and these were generally limited to dosing [40].

Free samples are not free. Although a short-course antibiotic may aid someone poor, samples increase the overall cost of medical care. The VHA and Kaiser Permanente recognize this fact and ban sample distribution [41]. Most samples are for chronic therapies that require a subsequent prescription. In the previously cited New York family practice study, if a prescription was written it was almost always for the same brand-name medication as the sample [39].

Brand loyalty to samples may balance treatment effects with increased costs.

Free samples do not begin to address the problem of the uninsured. Moreover, it is not fair to expect private shareholders to provide free care to the medically indigent. If physicians feel strongly that medical care is a public good then they might consider working for policy change that focuses on the taxpayer and not the strategic charity of pharmaceutical corporations.

Gifts: grants and publications

Industry support for research is primarily an economic investment. Common, even benign conditions attract dollars because they have the potential to generate significant revenue. Rare diseases, or those primarily afflicting third-world residents (tuberculosis, malaria, leishmaniasis) require "neglected" or "orphan" status to receive funding. For example, from 1975 to 1999, of the 1393 new drugs marketed, only 13, or less than 1%, were for tropical diseases [42]. Pharmaceutical firms focus on profitable areas to do research and marketing.

In addition, pharmaceutical funding is correlated with positive study results and inversely correlated with negative study results. One hundred seven controlled clinical trials, published in several respected internal medicine journals, were classified as either favoring a new, or traditional therapy. Seventy-one percent favored new therapies and 43% of these received pharmaceutical funding. Thirty-one trials supported traditional therapies, but only four (13%) were funded by industry. Tellingly, the sponsor's therapy was never deemed inferior to a treatment sold by another company [43]. Likewise, a study of 56 industry-supported nonsteroidal anti-inflammatory drugs, published in the late 1980s, reported the manufacturer's drug as comparable with (71.4%) or superior to (28.6%) the alternative drug in all trials [44]. From 1988 to 1998, a sample of the oncology literature revealed that company-sponsored studies were less likely than nonprofit-sponsored studies to report unfavorable qualitative conclusions (1 [5%] in 20 versus 9 [38%] in 24; $P = .04$) [45].

For those who lack writing skills or simply do not have adequate time to write, industry ghostwriters frequently produce proindustry articles published under the academic's name. Journals print these often unsolicited editorials coinciding with clinical developments or current controversies, with only bland admissions of drug company support [46]. Aside from the ethics involved in taking credit for another's work, the pseudoauthor often receives a gift worth $3000 or more, in addition to industry payments to the actual author. Parke-Davis called its marketing a "publications" strategy. It sponsored trivial research for off-label uses of gabapentin. Ghostwriters prepared articles and the company paid $12,000 for each of 12 articles. Afterward, academic "authors" were paid $1000 to sign them; a report to Parke-Davis complained, "Author interested; still playing phone tag" [28]. Then in caps, "(OUR FIRM) HAS DRAFT COMPLETE, WE JUST NEED AN AUTHOR" [47]. The articles are essentially infomercials for which only the pseudoauthor surgeon claims responsibility. Wrote one industry ghostwriter, "The way I look at it, if doctors have their name on it, that's their responsibility, not mine" [48].

Harm of accepting gifts

Loss of patient trust

The confidences people share with their attorneys, accountants, or ministers are not as deep as those divulged to their surgeon. Patients generally know that the nature of surgery confers a great risk of harm if truths are withheld. Patients provide their surgeons with accurate information, however, only if they completely trust that the practitioner's primary concern is their interest, and not self-interest [49].

Although a significant proportion of patients surveyed are unaware of industry gifts to physicians, patients ignorant of detailing were equally likely to harbor negative opinions about the effect of gifts on the cost and quality of health care [50]. Approximately one third of patients surveyed in a military facility understood the costs of gifts are passed-on to patients and 36% believed that acceptance of any gift obligates a physician to prescribe products from that company [36]. Still, the image of an altruistic medical profession might change when patients learn of detailing, and probably not for the better.

Loss of colleague's trust

Physicians trust themselves but not others, in part because of what their colleagues "are getting." For example, internal medicine residents surveyed in a West Coast United States program stated that industry promotions did not influence their own prescribing (61%), but only 16% believed other physicians were similarly unaffected [51]. One study found that 85% of medical students believe it is unethical for politicians to accept a gift, whereas only 46% found it improper to accept a gift of similar value themselves [52]. As residents, they typically receive more sponsored meals, whereas physicians in practice benefit from more honoraria, conference travel, and research funding [7]. They express concern that the information other doctors receive damages their coworkers objectivity [51].

Many physicians accept expensive gifts without reservation. In a recent survey of pharmaceutical detailing, internal medicine residents and faculty at a southeastern United States medical school judged various marketing practices as morally problematic or not. Textbooks worth $500, expensive meals, and $40 golf balls rated only "mildly problematic" for the residents (in this list only the golf balls approached "moderately problematic" for the faculty). Both groups agreed that an all-expense paid weekend trip to a resort hotel where the physician's only obligation is to spend several hours in seminars focusing on the company's products is "moderately problematic" [53]. Overall, the faculty seemed more reluctant to view gifts as innocuous, and the morality of lavish items was questioned by some.

Doctors' actions command the attention of other doctors. Respected physicians are often paid to promote at dinners and educational retreats. Some information is unbiased, but the industry does not pay (up to $2500 to chair roundtable discussions for rofecoxib) [54] if the message is unfriendly.

Irrational prescribing

Drug detailing is universally accompanied by gifts, and despite what many physicians believe, significantly affects prescribing habits. Advertising is effective. A 1987 survey of family physicians demonstrated that preference for prescribing brand-name medications, over their generic equivalents, strongly correlates with intensity of detailing, but was negatively correlated with readership of the *New England Journal of Medicine* [55]. Admittedly, the volume of advertising in almost all journals renders this reference standard suspect, but the authors imply that journal readers seek more objective sources than detailers, and the result is less brand-name medication usage. Moreover, family practitioners that relied more on pharmaceutical representative information had significantly increased prescription costs [56].

Examples of advertising's role in swaying clinicians toward lucrative rather than economic (or more appropriate) medications involved neuroprotective agents and analgesics. By the early 1980s, the medical literature clearly stated that propoxyphene analgesics were not superior to aspirin despite industry claims and drug detailing to the contrary. Similarly, company representatives (accompanied by gifts) continued to promote cerebral vasodilators as a treatment for senile dementia, although critical support was lacking. The result was that physicians kept prescribing the two drug classes long after published studies discounted both therapies, possibly indicating that many physicians were receiving their education from industrial sources, or were at least slow to adopt better practices in the presence of contradictory marketing [57].

Personal meetings with drug detailers are persuasive events, typically unrecorded, and likely filled with inaccuracies favorable to the drug or device for sale. In one study, 106 recorded statements by sales representatives at a university hospital contained 12 inaccuracies and all were favorable toward the promoted drug. None of 15 statements about the competitors' drugs were favorable; all of these were accurate, significantly ($P < .01$) differing from the fidelity of statements about the promoted drugs. Unfortunately, a minority (26%) of the 27 physicians who attended these presentations recalled a single false statement [58]. Because representatives were consented for the study, and aware that audio recordings were made of those talks, one might predict that standard, unobtrusive presentations contain significantly more biased statements. In this study all of the promoted drugs were patented with short-track records and competed with less expensive generics. One of the agents was even withdrawn from the market for excess mortality a scant 20 days after a talk promoting its use.

The frequency of formulary requests parallels advertising efforts. Forty physicians who requested a formulary addition from January 1989 through October 1990 at a United States university hospital were compared with 80 control physicians; the former were fivefold more likely to have accepted money from companies to attend or speak at educational symposia (95% CI 2–13.2) [59]. Furthermore, formulary requests after meetings with detailers were specific for those companies at a rate 13-fold the control group (95% CI 4.8–36.3) [59]. Advertising is effective, but its costs are reflected in increasing prices of medication and services.

Extreme advertising or gifting is extremely effective. Trips to luxury resorts attract media attention because the potential for bias is obvious. Still, 10 participants in all-expense-paid vacations believed that such enticements would not alter their prescribing patterns. Despite this belief, the usage of drug A (a new intravenous antibiotic) increased from a mean of 81 $\pm$ 44 units before the symposium to a mean of 272 ± 117 after the symposium ($P<.001$), and the usage of drug B (a new intravenous cardiovascular drug) changed from 34 ± 30 units to 87 ± 24 ($P<.001$) [60].

Detailing exists only for profitable, patented treatments. Some of these are true breakthrough medications and devices, but many compete with older, cheaper treatments that are equally, or more, effective (aspirin, hydrochlorothiazide, β-blockers), and possibly safer. For example, rofecoxib, trovafloxacin mesylate, and cerivastatin sodium representatives paid for thousands of lunches, talks, and distributed millions of toys and pens; these products were all subsequently restricted or eliminated for excess mortality. In these instances, individuals and society pay for overpriced medications and services. Marginal gains in efficacy, reduction in undesired side effects, or dosing simplicity are extolled in spectacular advertising campaigns and floods of sample packs. Toys, treats, books, gadgets, dinners, and trips foster a carnival atmosphere. For instance, attendees at the national emergency medicine conference in Seattle, 2002, received tote bags of toys on the exhibition floor while lined-up for steak from the manufacturer of the heart-drug eptifibatide.

The doctor-patient relationship

The hazard self-interest poses to a surgeon's fiduciary role is mostly navigable by applying general medical ethical codes of conduct. The principles taught to first-year medical students (nonmaleficence, beneficence, and honesty) serve as an invaluable guide to surgeon interactions with detailers [35]. The bottom line, however, is that surgeons and physicians have a duty to expend patients' health care resources wisely and honestly, using their best judgment, devoid of self-interest.

Nonmaleficence

Doing no harm to patients assumes that medical information is the best possible. The fact that there is serious reason to dispute the veracity of detailers' advertising claims has been presented. The harmful effect is difficult to measure, but very real. One example is the cost inflation of medical care, inflated by marketing efforts. Patent-protection is a two-edged sword. It provides strong stimulus for development and helps drive market success. Patents, however, inflate drug charges. Comparing the price of a drug once it becomes generic (eg, loratadine and omeprazole) with the drug's cost during its last year under patent illustrates a disconnect between production costs and final price. Increases in medical costs likely reduce the quantity, or quality, of care delivered. Nonmaleficence directs practitioners to minimize costs without compromising care.

Beneficence

Beneficence is the desire to help others. Accepting gifts is the desire to help oneself. At issue is whether these are mutually exclusive. History and contemporary media are critical of politicians accepting lobbyists' gifts and suspicion of surgeon kickbacks cannot be far behind. Although a token gift does not destroy a physician's integrity, the perception of inappropriate self-interest, or at least self-deception, weighs against beneficent behavior and the practitioner's character [19,35].

Veracity and honesty

Truth-telling and honesty are vital aspects to earn and maintain patient trust. They rely on their surgeons and physicians to act as their fiduciaries, steering them to the proper course of therapy based on scientific evidence and their sound judgment. Violating, or appearing to violate, that trust may be the most damaging part of the entire surgeon-industry gift-promotion dance. Society holds clinicians to a very high standard; even appearing to violate it damages clinicians as individual professionals and the entire medical community.

Summary

Why does gifting exist in the medical marketplace? It provides a sales advantage in a competitive marketplace by establishing crucial relationships with the patients' fiduciary: the physician and surgeon.

Do gifts to physicians from industry harm patients? One can cite mountains of indirect evidence that they do, and maybe in the case of recalled devices and drugs there are actual corpses, but these examples are retrospective and it is impossible to prove that removing detailing eliminates the harm.

Banning gifts to surgeons would not completely fix the ethical problem of pharmaceutical and device marketing. Gifts are important because they buy access and foster relationships, but inherent bias in research and the medical literature makes it very difficult to remain objective. It is a race, and education has not kept pace with advertising; only 10% of 575 internal medicine physicians thought they had

had sufficient training during medical school and residency regarding professional interaction with sales representatives [2].

Would banning gifts help at all? Would enforcing an unpopular ethical code protect patients? There might be a small improvement, but not as significant as eliminating representatives and product samples altogether. This is not likely to happen without an enormous fight against the wealthiest industry in America.

The solution is education. To borrow industry's argument, physicians and surgeons are ethical creatures with capacity for judgment and integrity. They need to understand and believe the magnitude of the problem. Detailing exists because there is a market for it, empowering surgeons with ethical training reduces the demand for goodies, and at some point the popular choice will be to buy their own lunch.

Business ethics are not medical ethics. Industry is behaving exactly as it must to maximize profits. Although it is painful for some surgeons, surgical residencies, and professional organizations to envision a future with diminished corporate gifts, it is every surgeon's responsibility to consider whether their dealings with the pharmaceutical and medical equipment industries withstand the harsh light of realities presented herein.

References

[1] Allman R. The relationship between physicians and the pharmaceutical industry: ethical problems with the every-day conflict of interest. HEC Forum 2003;15: 155–70.

[2] McKinney W, Schiedermayer D, Lurie N, et al. Attitudes of internal medicine faculty and residents toward professional interaction with pharmaceutical sales representatives. JAMA 1990;264:1693–7.

[3] Wilkes M. New York Times Magazine November 5, 1989;88–93.

[4] Jones L. Drug firms urged curb promotional gifts. Am Med News December 28, 1990;33(48):1.

[5] Bowman M, Pearle D. Changes in drug prescribing patterns related to commercial company funding of continuing medical education. J Contin Educ Health Prof 1988;8:13–20.

[6] Sales forces, scripts up in 1999. Pharmaceutical Representative. Northfield (IL): Publisher Advanstar Communications. Accessed September 21, 2001.

[7] Wazana A. Physicians and the pharmaceutical industry: is a gift ever just a gift? JAMA 2000;283:373–80.

[8] Blumenthal D. Doctors and drug companies. N Engl J Med 2004;351:1885–90.

[9] Relman A, Angell M. America's other drug problem. The New Republic 2002;227(25):27–41.

[10] Szabo L. Health systems cutting costs by closing door on drug reps. USA Today August 25, 2004;12B.

[11] Hodges B. Interactions with the pharmaceutical industry. CMAJ 1995;153:553–9.

[12] Access is worth its wait in gold. Repertoire 2003; 11(10). http://www.medicaldistribution.com/rep/Rep_2003_October/toc.htm.

[13] Spilker B. The benefits and risks of a pack of M&Ms: a pharmaceutical spokesman answers his industry's critics. Health Aff (Millwood) 2002;21:243–4.

[14] Spilker B. The benefits and risks of a pack of M&Ms: a pharmaceutical spokesman answers his industry's critics. Health Aff (Millwood) 2002;21:298–9.

[15] Committee on Labor and Human Resources. Marketing, and promotional practices of the pharmaceutical industry. Washington: US Government Printing Office; 1991.

[16] Bricker E. Industrial marketing and medical ethics. N Engl J Med 1989;320:1690–2.

[17] American Medical Association. Opinion E-8.061: clarifying addendum, 2004. Available at: http://www.ama-assn.org/ama/pub/category/4263.html. Accessed February 4, 2005.

[18] Orentlicher D. Gifts to physicians from industry. JAMA 1991;265:501.

[19] Goldfinger S. Physicians and the pharmaceutical industry. Ann Intern Med 1990;112:624–6.

[20] Department of Veterans Health Affairs. Business relationships between VHA staff and pharmaceutical industry representatives. VHA directive 2003–060. Washington: US Government Printing Office; 2003.

[21] Goodman B. No free lunch. Available at: http://www.nofreelunch.org. Accessed November 24, 2004.

[22] Rogers W, Mansfield P, Braunack-Mayer A. The ethics of pharmaceutical industry relationships with medical students. Med J Aust 2004;180:411–4.

[23] Studdert D, Mello M, Brennan T. Financial conflicts of interest in physicians' relationships with the pharmaceutical industry self-regulation in the shadow of federal prosecution. N Engl J Med 2004;351: 1891–900.

[24] Harris G. Guilty plea seen for drug maker. New York Times July 16, 2004;1,4.

[25] Harris G. As doctor writes prescription, drug company writes a check. New York Times June 27, 2004;1,1.

[26] Ross B, Scott D. Influencing doctors: how pharmaceutical companies use enticement to "educate" physicians (ABCnews.com), 2002. Available at: http://www.vaccinationnews.com/DailyNews?February2002/InfluencingDoctors.htm. Accessed February 21, 2002.

[27] Department of Health and Human Services OIG. OIG compliance program guidance for pharmaceutical manufacturers. Federal Register 2003;68:23731–43.

[28] Relman A. Defending professional independence: ACCME's proposed new guidelines for commercial support of CME. JAMA 2003;289:2418–20.

[29] Macneil I. Exchange revisited: individual utility and social solidarity. Ethics 1986;96:657–93.

[30] Belk R. It's the thought that counts: a signed digraph analysis of gift-giving. J Consum Res 1976;3:155–62.

[31] Sherry J. Gift giving in anthropological perspective. J Consum Res 1983;10:157–67.
[32] Coyle S. Physician-industry relations. Part 1: Individual physicians. Ann Intern Med 2002;136:396–402.
[33] Randall T. Ethics of receiving gifts considered. JAMA 1991;265:442–3.
[34] Blake RJ, Early E. Patients' attitudes about gifts to physicians from pharmaceutical companies. J Am Board Fam Pract 1995;8:457–64.
[35] Chren M, Landefeld C, Murray T. Doctors, drug companies, and gifts. JAMA 1989;262:3448–51.
[36] Gibbons R, Landry F, Blouch D. A comparison of physicians' and patients' attitudes toward pharmaceutical industry gifts. J Gen Intern Med 1998;13:151–4.
[37] Peay M, Peay E. The role of commercial sources in the adoption of a new drug. Soc Sci Med 1988;26:1183–9.
[38] Shaughnessy A, Bucci K. Drug samples and family practice residents. Ann Pharmacother 1997;31:1296–300.
[39] Morelli D, Koenigsberg M. Sample medication dispensing in a residency practice. J Fam Pract 1992;34:42–8.
[40] Backer E, Lebsack J, Reiner J. The value of pharmaceutical representative visits and medication samples in community-based family practices. J Fam Pract 2000;49:811–6.
[41] Vrazo F. Hospitals get tough with drug firm reps (Philadelphia Inquirer). Available at: http://www.philly.com/mld/inquirer/9964610.htm?1c. Accessed November 22, 2004.
[42] Banerji J. The gap is growing: more resources needed now for neglected diseases. Available at: http://www.dndi.org/cms/public_html/insidearticleListing.asp?CategoryId=166&SubCategoryId=167&ArticleId=315&TemplateId=1. Accessed November 22, 2004.
[43] Davidson R. Source of funding and outcome of clinical trials. J Gen Intern Med 1986;1:155–8.
[44] Rochon P, Gurwitz J, Simms R. A study of manufacturer-supported trials of nonsteroidal anti-inflammatory drugs in the treatment of arthritis. Arch Intern Med 1994;154:157–63.
[45] Friedberg M, Saffran B, Stinson T, et al. Evaluation of conflict of interest in economic analyses of new drugs used in oncology. JAMA 1999;282:1453–7.
[46] Brennan T. Sounding board: buying editorials. N Engl J Med 1994;331:673–5.
[47] Ross J, Lurie P, Wolfe S. Concepts in professional education and communications. Why should you invest in medical education? Available at: http://www.citizen.org/publications/release.cfm?ID=6731. Accessed March 11, 2005.
[48] Johnson E, Jones C. Inside the business of medical ghostwriting (CBC News). Available at: http://www.cbc.ca/story/science/national/2002/10/24/drug_res021024.html. Accessed November 24, 2004.
[49] Sade R. Profits and professionalism. J Thorac Cardiovasc Surg 2002;123:403–5.
[50] Mainous A, Hueston W, Rich E. Patient perceptions of physician acceptance of gifts from the pharmaceutical industry. Arch Fam Med 1995;4:335–9.
[51] Steinman M, Shlipak M, McPhee S. Of principles and pens: attitudes and practices of medicine house staff toward pharmaceutical industry promotions. Am J Med 2001;110:551–7.
[52] Palmisano P, Edelstein J. Teaching drug promotion abuses to health profession students. J Med Educ 1980;55:453–5.
[53] Brett A, Burr W, Moloo J. Are gifts from pharmaceutical companies ethically problematic? Arch Intern Med 2003;163:2213–8.
[54] Barry P. Prescription drugs–the insiders. AARP Bulletin November 2004;10–5.
[55] Bower A, Burkett G. Family physicians and generic drugs: a study of recognition, information sources, prescribing attitudes, and practices. J Fam Pract 1987;24:612–6.
[56] Caudill T, Johnson M, Rich E, et al. Physicians, pharmaceutical sales representatives, and the cost of prescribing. Arch Fam Med 1996;5:201–6.
[57] Avorn J, Chen M, Hartley R. Scientific versus commercial sources of influence on the prescribing behavior of physicians. Am J Med 1982;73:4–8.
[58] Ziegler M, Lew P, Singer B. The accuracy of drug information from pharmaceutical sales representatives. JAMA 1995;273:1296–8.
[59] Chren M, Landefeld C. Physicians' behavior and their interactions with drug companies: a controlled study of physicians who requested additions to a hospital formulary. JAMA 1994;271:684–9.
[60] Orlowski J, Wateska L. The effects of pharmaceutical firm enticements on physician prescribing patterns: there's no such thing as a free lunch. Chest 1992;102:270–3.

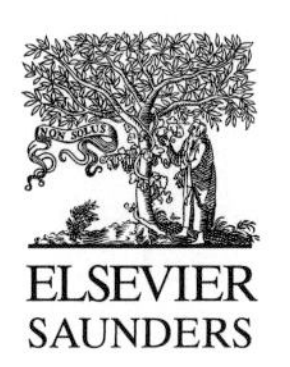
ELSEVIER
SAUNDERS

Thorac Surg Clin 15 (2005) 543 – 554

THORACIC
SURGERY
CLINICS

Ethical Issues in Surgical Research

Franklin G. Miller, PhD

Department of Clinical Bioethics, Clinical Center, National Institutes of Health, Building 10, Room 1C118, Bethesda, MD 20892–1156, USA

Surgical research poses a variety of distinctive ethical challenges, in addition to sharing those that are common to research in other medical domains. This article focuses on ethical issues that have a particular salience in surgical research. Topics examined include (1) the prevalence of surgical procedures that have not been rigorously evaluated in randomized controlled trials (RCTs); (2) the unclear boundary between innovative surgical practice and research; (3) control group selection in surgical trials, with particular attention to sham surgery controls; and (4) issues of informed consent. To set the stage for addressing the latter two topics, the importance of distinguishing the ethics of clinical research from the ethics of clinical care is examined in some detail.

Research on the efficacy of surgical procedures

For more than 40 years, commentators have lamented the fact that new surgical procedures are introduced into practice and maintained as standard therapies without rigorous efficacy evaluation. In a classic article concerning the placebo effect of surgery, Beecher [1] observed that "One may question the moral or ethical right to continue with casual or unplanned new surgical procedures—procedures which may encompass no more than a placebo effect—when these procedures are costly of time and money, and dangerous to health or life." The most frequent method of efficacy research in surgery has been the retrospective case series, which presents data on outcomes relating to surgical procedures without any comparison with a concurrent control group [2,3]. The data from such uncontrolled studies may suffice to establish the effectiveness of new surgical procedures when the natural history of the disease is well understood and objective outcomes are dramatic, as in the case of antiseptic techniques, removing a ruptured appendix, or organ transplantation [4]. If benefits in reduced mortality or morbidity are less substantial or not clearly attributable to the specific surgical procedure, however, data from case series provide, at best, weak evidence of efficacy. This type of research is subject to systematic biases and is not designed to counteract the fallacy of post hoc ergo propter hoc: observed benefit following surgery does not imply that the surgical procedure caused the improvement. When well-designed RCTs have been conducted, various established surgical procedures have been found to have an unfavorable risk-benefit ratio or to be no more effective than a placebo intervention. These include experimental evaluation of internal mammary artery ligation to treat angina [5,6], extracranial-intracranial bypass operation to prevent strokes [7], arthroscopic surgery for osteoarthritis of the knee [8], and adenotonsillectomy for children with throat infections [9]. In sum, the introduction and maintenance of surgical procedures without sufficiently rigorous efficacy evaluation poses undue risks of harm to patients and is contrary to evidence-based practice.

Various reasons account for the relative paucity of RCTs in surgery as compared with other medical specialties. Probably most important is the fact that the US Food and Drug Administration does not regulate surgical procedures. Whereas the law mandates that new pharmaceutical agents cannot be in-

The opinions expressed are those of the author and do not necessarily reflect the position or policy of the National Institutes of Health, the Public Health Service, or the Department of Health and Human Services.

E-mail address: fmiller@nih.gov

1547-4127/05/$ – see front matter. Published by Elsevier Inc.
doi:10.1016/j.thorsurg.2005.06.008

troduced into clinical practice without prior rigorous efficacy evaluation, surgical procedures are not subject to prospective regulation for safety and efficacy external to prevailing professional standards. Moreover, pharmaceutical and biotechnology companies generally have little or no commercial interest in the development of innovative surgical procedures, substantially reducing financial support for RCTs.

The culture of surgery may also contribute to avoiding RCTs [10]. The design and conduct of RCTs are predicated both scientifically and ethically on a state of uncertainty regarding the therapeutic merits of new or existing treatments. The practice of surgery, however, because it involves invasive procedures, demands an activist orientation, characterized by confidence and decisiveness in practitioners. This spirit is captured by the surgical motto "sometimes in error, never in doubt" [11]. Convinced of their ability to benefit patients by means of surgical intervention, surgeons may be reluctant to test the efficacy of their procedures in RCTs. Moreover, this propensity to therapeutic conviction gives rise to the dubious stance that it is unethical to withhold established or innovative surgical procedures in RCTs comparing them with standard medical treatment.

Finally, various practical problems impede the conduct of RCTs in surgery [3,12]. The learning curve for developing innovative procedures, the incremental evolution of technique, and the importance of experience to successful outcomes make it more difficult to standardize surgical procedures for rigorous evaluation, as compared with pharmaceutical treatments. Complete masking of treatment assignment for the research team is impossible, because the surgeon must know the operation being performed. It is difficult to keep patient-subjects in the dark about whether they are receiving a particular surgical intervention without the use of placebo or sham operations, which raise serious ethical issues discussed in detail later. In view of the invasiveness of surgery, patients may be reluctant to submit to random assignment of surgery or a medical treatment. Nonetheless, these practical difficulties do not preclude the rigorous design and conduct of RCTs of surgical procedures.

The boundary between innovative practice and research

The development of innovative surgical procedures without formal, rigorous evaluation has meant that patients are often exposed to experimental interventions without oversight by institutional review boards under federal regulations governing research with human subjects and without adequate informed consent. Determining when surgical innovation constitutes research is not clear-cut [13]. The Belmont Report, developed in 1979 by the National Commission for the Protection of Human Subjects of Biomedical and Behavioral Research to formulate ethical principles and guidelines for the protection of human subjects of research, described the boundary between practice and research in the following way [14]:

> For the most part, the term "practice" refers to interventions that are designed solely to enhance the well-being of an individual patient or client and that have a reasonable expectation of success. The purpose of medical or behavioral practice is to provide diagnosis, preventive treatment, or therapy to particular individuals. By contrast, the term "research" designates an activity designed to test a hypothesis, permit conclusions to be drawn, and thereby to develop or contribute to generalizable knowledge.... When a clinician departs in a significant way from standard or accepted practice, the innovation does not, in and of itself, constitute research.... Radically new procedures of this description should, however, be made the object of formal research at an early stage to determine whether they are safe and effective.

Innovations introduced into the context of clinical practice become research at least at the point that the results are written up for publication in a retrospective case series [15]. Reitsma and Moreno [16] reported pilot data on the extent to which the results of surgical innovation described in published articles had received institutional review board review. A search of United States surgical and medical journals yielded 59 articles published between 1992 and 2000 that described surgical innovation. Questionnaires were sent to study authors. Only 21 questionnaires were returned; however, the results are suggestive. Although 14 authors described their reported innovative procedures as research, only 6 had sought prior institutional review board review. The respondents indicated that informed consent documents described the innovative nature of the procedure in only 6 out of the 21 cases. Accordingly, the current practice of surgical innovation seems to reflect a disposition to have it both ways: to experiment with innovative surgical procedures within the informal framework of clinical care and without institutional review board oversight at the same time as publishing research based on surgical innovation in professional journals. As Margo [15] has aptly observed, "Although preliminary surgical studies are imperfect, they need to be conducted openly and not disguised as clinical care then later reported as a retrospective series." Both the quality of research and the protection of patient-subjects are likely to be enhanced by developing formal research protocols for surgical innovation and submitting them to institutional review board review.

Distinguishing clinical research and clinical care

Although the boundary between innovative surgery and research may be difficult to draw in particular cases, the distinction between practice and research, outlined by the Belmont Report, is central to developing a sound ethical framework for clinical research in general and surgical research in particular [17]. Clinical care has a personalized focus. It is directed to helping a particular person in need of expert medical attention. Clinical research essentially lacks this purpose of personalized help for particular individuals. Contrary to what the definition of "research" in the Belmont Report might suggest, what makes clinical research distinctive is not the testing of a hypothesis or permitting conclusions to be drawn. The practice of medicine necessarily involves physicians formulating and testing diagnostic hypotheses to draw conclusions about what is wrong with a particular patient, which then lead to decisions about the appropriate treatment to recommend. The same point can be made about the term "experimentation," which is often taken as a synonym for research. Clinical care typically involves experimentation in the process of finding treatments that work for a given patient and adjusting them so that therapeutic benefit can be maximized and side effects or complications minimized. Rather, it is the aim of producing generalizable knowledge by means of experimentation with, or observation of, human subjects that distinguishes clinical research. Clinical research is primarily concerned with investigating defined groups of subjects, in contrast to the focus of clinical care on individual patients. In sum, the purpose of inviting individuals to participate in clinical research primarily is not to help them but to develop generalizable knowledge about diseases and their treatment that can be used to help others in the future.

The distinctive purpose of clinical research, which makes it an essentially different activity from clinical care, gives rise to the use of characteristic methods that are foreign to medical care. These include such procedures as random assignment of treatments, the use of placebo controls, and techniques to mask treatments so that subjects, and often investigators, do not know what treatment they are receiving. In addition, scientific protocols governing clinical trials typically restrict flexibility in adjusting doses of study drugs and using concomitant treatments. The ethical significance of these research methods is that research subjects are required to forgo the individualized attention characteristic of clinical care, in which treatments are selected to be optimal for them, and both patient and doctor know what treatment is being received. Instead, clinical trial participants are treated according to a protocol designed to generate scientifically valid data.

The distinctive purpose of clinical research to develop generalizable knowledge leads to another key difference relating to the justification of risks. In clinical care, risks of diagnostic procedures and treatments are justified by potential medical benefits to the patients who receive them. There is an important exception in the domain of surgery in the case of organ transplantation involving living donors, in which the risks to one patient are justified by the benefits to another. But this does not change the pervasive orientation of medical and surgical practice to seeking proportionality between risks and benefits for the particular patient seeking clinical care. In clinical research, the risks of some interventions, such as experimental treatments, may be justified, at least in part, by the prospect of benefit to individual subjects. Nearly all clinical research, however, includes one or more procedures that carry burdens or risks to individual subjects without any compensating medical benefits to them. In some studies the entire set of procedures involving human subjects falls into this nonbeneficial category. Randomized clinical trials, which evaluate treatments for patient-subjects diagnosed with a given condition, typically include interventions to measure study outcomes, such as blood draws, biopsies, lumbar punctures, and imaging procedures. These procedures are necessary to generate scientifically valid data but do not provide any medical benefit to research subjects.

Confusing research and care

Despite the clear differences between clinical research and clinical care in purpose, methods, and justification of risks, it remains easy to confuse the two activities in the concrete circumstances in which clinical research takes place [17]. Clinical research is conducted by physicians in hospitals and increasingly in doctors' offices. Investigators and members of the research team wear white coats. Instruments and procedures commonly used in clinical care are also used for research purposes. In addition, the language used to describe clinical research contributes to confusion. Subjects are often referred to as "patients" and investigators as "doctors," without any qualifiers indicating that an activity distinct from clinical care is being pursued. Clinical trials are often described as "therapeutic research," and investigators as having a "therapeutic intent." The website for M.D. Anderson, a leading cancer research and care center, asserts that "A clinical trial is just one of many treatment options at M.D. Anderson," [18] suggesting that the scientific experimentation of clinical trials is a form of medical therapy.

These factors produce or reinforce a tendency observed in patient-subjects to conflate research participation and medical care, a phenomenon known as "the therapeutic misconception" [19]. Patients enrolled in clinical trials often see their participation as defined by the same personalized patient-centered orientation characteristic of medical care. Investigators also may harbor therapeutic misconceptions about the ethics of clinical research.

Moreover, ethical thinking about clinical research also displays a misguided therapeutic orientation. The idea that physicians are devoted to the health and well-being of their patients is so deeply ingrained that it is difficult to grasp that in clinical research conducted by physicians in clinical settings the primary obligation of investigators is not to promote the health and well-being of patients enrolled in research. Instead, investigators must protect research subjects from exploitation and undue risks of harm. The conflation between the ethics of clinical research and the ethics of clinical medicine is notably manifested in the Declaration of Helsinki, which stipulates "ethical principles for medical research involving human subjects" [20]. Principle number 3 states, "The Declaration of Geneva of the World Medical Association binds the physician with the words, 'The health of my patient will be my first consideration.'" This is certainly a sound principle for the ethics of therapeutic medicine; however, its appearance in the leading international code of ethics for clinical research is puzzling. It implies that clinical research should be governed by the patient-centered therapeutic beneficence characteristic of medical care. Most clinical research would be impossible to conduct if it were strictly governed by the ethical framework appropriate to clinical care.

Clinical equipoise

The prevailing ethical thinking about clinical trials, which invokes the principle of "clinical equipoise," has endeavored to justify these scientific experiments in the context of the therapeutic physician-patient relationship. According to this principle, a clinical trial is ethical only if the expert medical community is uncertain about the relative therapeutic merits of the experimental and control treatments evaluated in the trial [21]. When a state of clinical equipoise exists, no patient is randomized to a treatment known to be inferior to available therapeutic options, making clinical trials compatible with the therapeutic obligation of physicians. Freedman and colleagues [22] assert that "As a normative matter, it [clinical equipoise] defines ethical trial design as prohibiting any compromise of a patient's right to medical treatment by enrolling in a study." According to the principle of clinical equipoise it is wrong to randomize a trial participant to a placebo control when proved effective treatment is available for the participant's medical condition. Clinical equipoise "foreclose[s] the use of placebos in the face of established treatment, because enrolling in a trial would imply that a proportion of enrollees will receive medical attention currently considered inferior by the expert community" [22].

Clinical equipoise was proposed as a solution to an ethical problem known as "the RCT dilemma": how is it possible to conduct randomized trials enrolling patients in need of medical treatment without violating the therapeutic obligation of physicians to promote the medical best interests of patients [23]. Gifford [24] described this dilemma as follows:

> The central dilemma concerning randomized clinical trials (RCTs) arises out of some simple facts about causal methodology (RCTs are the best way to generate the reliable causal knowledge necessary for optimally-informed action) and a prima facie plausible principle concerning how physicians should treat their patients (always do what it is most reasonable to believe will be best for the patient).

In view of the distinction between clinical research and medical care, this amounts to a spurious dilemma [23]. That physicians should have undivided loyalty to do what they believe is best medically for their patients is certainly a plausible principle for clinical care. It is not a plausible principle for governing the relationship between investigators and research subjects. Because the clinical trial should be conceived as a controlled experiment aimed to evaluate treatments scientifically, rather than as a form of personalized medical therapy, it is difficult to see why the therapeutic obligation of physicians or the right of patients to optimal medical care must govern thinking about the ethics of randomized trials. Specifically, it is difficult to see why in the context of research it is wrong per se to provide less than optimal or standard treatment in the form of a placebo control. Use of a placebo may be wrong because it is not methodologically necessary for a valid test of the study hypothesis or because withholding treatment or the use of an invasive sham operation is likely to cause serious harm. Yet, to see it as wrong because it compromises the patient's right to medical treatment conflates research with therapy.

Ethical problems with the therapeutic orientation

What is wrong from an ethical perspective with the therapeutic orientation to clinical research [17]? First, it produces false moral comfort about clinical research. Using some for the good of others is inherent in clinical research. The therapeutic orientation makes it seem that in pursuing research investigators are maintaining their therapeutic obligations to patient-subjects. This distorts the moral climate and diverts attention from the potential for exploitation in the research enterprise. Second, the therapeutic orientation may contribute to subtle exploitation insofar as it encourages investigators to use their authority as physicians to secure participation in research, an activity that is not aimed at the best interests of subjects. This is of greatest concern when there is a prior therapeutic relationship between the physician-investigator and the prospective research subject.

Third, the therapeutic orientation to research interferes with the development of a proper sense of professional integrity among investigators [25]. Integrity involves coherence between beliefs and conduct. Unlike clinical care, clinical trials typically include procedures designed to generate valid scientific data, which are known to pose risks to subjects that are not compensated by potential benefits to them (eg, a biopsy performed solely to measure study outcomes). When physician-investigators see patient volunteers and themselves in the guise of the therapeutic physician-patient relationship, while they conduct research activities that depart significantly from the ethical framework of clinical care, their professional self-understanding lacks integrity.

Fourth, the therapeutic orientation interferes with informed consent to participate in research. Patients have not consented to research if they think of it simply as therapy. It is likely that a therapeutic orientation to research by investigators fosters the therapeutic misconception among patient volunteers. If investigators view the ethics of clinical research through a therapeutic lens, how can one expect research subjects to be clear about how their participation in research differs from the context of clinical care? Finally, the therapeutic orientation fails to provide adequate guidance regarding what types of clinical trials are ethically acceptable. As illustrated later, this perspective on the ethics of clinical research has led to a categorical opposition to the use of placebo controls in surgical research.

An ethical framework appropriate to clinical research

It might be objected that the effort to distinguish the ethics of clinical research from the ethics of medical care is bound to leave research subjects without adequate protection. It invites rampant exploitation under a utilitarian ethic, which sanctions sacrificing the well-being of research subjects for the sake of scientific progress. The claim that research ethics is not properly governed by therapeutic norms does not imply, however, that there are no ethical constraints on scientific investigation to protect research participants from harm and exploitation.

Emanuel and coworkers [26] explicate seven ethical requirements of clinical research, drawing in part on the Belmont Report. These requirements include (1) that research projects aim at socially valuable health-related knowledge; (2) that rigorous methods are used to produce scientifically valid data; (3) that subjects are selected fairly; (4) that research protocols have a favorable risk-benefit ratio, which involves minimizing risks and justifying them by the prospect of medical benefits to research subjects or the value of knowledge to be gained; (5) that research protocols receive independent committee review and oversight; (6) that informed consent is obtained; and (7) that enrolled research participants are treated with respect during the course of research. These requirements can, and should, be understood in a way that does not imply that research is governed by the ethics of therapeutic medicine. Together they provide the grounds for robust protection of human subjects while permitting valuable research to proceed. This ethical framework provides valuable guidance for assessing controversial issues in the design and conduct of clinical research, including the topic of sham surgery discussed in the next section.

Control group selection: sham surgery

Randomized placebo-controlled trials are widely considered to be the most rigorous method of evaluating treatment efficacy. From a methodologic perspective, sham-controlled surgery trials are particularly valuable when the outcome measures are based on inherently subjective reports of patients, such as pain, symptom improvement, and quality of life. Because of ethical concerns, however, there have been very few randomized clinical trials comparing a new or standard surgery with a sham surgery control.

The leading ethical arguments against the use of sham surgery in randomized clinical trials are based on faulty reasoning [27]. These arguments involve three mistakes: (1) confusing the ethics of clinical research with the ethics of clinical medicine; (2) taking a single controversial case (fetal tissue transplantation for Parkinson's disease) as paradigmatic of sham surgery without carefully considering the possibility that less risky sham surgery controls may present a favorable research risk-benefit ratio; and (3) misinterpreting the ethical requirement for clinical research of minimizing risks.

Conflating the ethics of clinical research with the ethics of clinical care

The purpose of using any placebo control in a double-blind randomized clinical trial, including sham surgery, is to mimic the experience of receiving a specific treatment, so as to seem indistinguishable to patient volunteers from the real treatment that is being evaluated rigorously. Typically, pill placebos are inert substances, which carry no risks in themselves but may pose significant risks from withholding standard treatment. In contrast, sham surgery is an invasive placebo control that carries the risks of the fake operation and concomitant treatment, such as anesthesia.

The prospect of using a sham surgery in a clinical trial is likely to evoke an intuitive judgment that this is unethical. Summarizing the literature on surgical research, Frader and Caniano [28] report:

> One can find only a few supporters in the mid-1990s for placebo or what have been called sham controls in surgical research. One text states baldly "...sham operations are ethically unjustifiable and would not be considered today." Another group states a similar position, "The only true placebo is a sham operation which is unethical. Surgical trials cannot, therefore, be fully placebo controlled."

The reasoning in support of this blanket rejection of sham surgery might be formulated as follows. Surgeons have the license and the privilege to cut into the live human body for the sake of healing. Accordingly, to use surgical instruments to perform a fake operation as a control patently violates the basic moral imperative of medical ethics: do no harm. As a rule, physicians should not expose patients to risks from interventions unless they are reasonably believed by competent practitioners to be outweighed by potential medical benefits. Surgeons and other physicians do not cease being bound by the basic norms of medical ethics when they undertake clinical trials. In an extended critique of sham surgery, Clark [29] asserts:

> The researcher has an ethical responsibility to act in the best interest of subjects. The belief that a particular clinical trial will not cause too much harm to too many people or that society will benefit at the possible expense of particular individuals violates the duty of the researcher to act in the best interest of the subject. To determine whether that duty has been breached, a researcher's actions should be measured against the accepted standard of practice as set by professional norms.

Judged by the surgical standard of care, use of sham surgery is unethical, because conscientious surgeons do not perform fake operations or undertake surgery unless they judge it to be in the best medical interests of patients. As London and Kadane [30] observe, "Using a sham surgery component in the control again adds risks of foreseeable and preventable harm without a corresponding benefit to subjects in the control arm. As a result, it is difficult to see how the use of sham surgery controls might be reconciled with the duty of personal care."

This moral stance, which makes sham surgery seem inherently or presumptively unethical, adopts the therapeutic orientation to clinical research and confuses the ethics of clinical research with the ethics of clinical care [17,23]. The ethically significant differences between clinical research and medical care described previously (differences in purpose, methods, and justification of risks) imply that it is erroneous to hold that clinical research should be governed by the same ethical standards as apply to the practice of medicine. Indeed, by its very nature, the RCT departs from the duty of personal care. Sham surgery is not unethical just because it exposes patients to risks that are not compensated by medical benefits. Sham surgery as a control should be evaluated in terms of the ethical requirements proper to clinical research.

Three cases of sham surgery

The ethical commentary over sham surgery has concentrated on the evaluation of fetal tissue transplantation in the treatment of Parkinson's disease

[29–36]. The use of aborted human fetal tissue and the nature of the sham procedure, which involved drilling holes in the skull, make the controversial research intervention of sham surgery seem all the more ethically dubious. Expanding the ethical focus to reflect on two other important cases promotes a more balanced assessment of sham surgery.

Internal mammary artery ligation

Ligation of the internal mammary artery to treat angina became a widely adopted surgery in the 1950s [1]. At the end of that decade the results of two sham-controlled trials to evaluate this procedure were reported in the medical literature, both of which demonstrated that it was no better than a sham operation involving skin incision under local anesthesia without ligation of the internal mammary artery [5,6]. Ligation of the internal mammary artery was abandoned in the wake of the published results, indicating the potential power of sham-controlled trials to influence clinical practice and protect patients from risky procedures without specific efficacy beyond the placebo effect.

These sham-controlled trials were conducted without fully informed consent from the patient-subjects. Cobb and coworkers [5] in their report noted, "The patients were told only that they were participating in an evaluation of this operation; they were not informed of the double-blind nature of the study." They were not informed that they might receive a sham operation rather than the real surgery. Despite lack of informed consent, which was consistent with research practice at the time [37], this study remains valuable in thinking about the methodologic rationale and risk-benefit assessment for sham surgery.

Fetal tissue transplantation

The contemporary ethical debate has centered on controversial sham-controlled trials involving transplantation of fetal neural tissue into the brains of patients with severe Parkinson's disease. Based on promising results of preclinical animal studies and open, uncontrolled trials of fetal tissue transplantation, the National Institutes of Health sponsored two placebo-controlled trials. One of these trials has been the focus of considerable ethical attention, prompted by a "Sounding Board" article in *The New England Journal of Medicine*, which described the research in detail and defended it on methodologic and ethical grounds [31].

The sham control arm of this trial was designed to present to patients the same experience of the fetal tissue transplantation procedure and postprocedure treatment without injecting an inert substance into the brains of patients randomized to the sham control. It carried substantial risks for patient volunteers. These included a slight risk of death from general anesthesia; and discomfort and possible complications from the placing of stereotactic equipment on the skull, scalp incisions, and the drilling of burr holes, which did not penetrate the dura. To maintain the blind conditions of the trial, those patients randomized to the sham intervention also were given low doses of cyclosporine, provided as an immunosuppressive treatment for the patients receiving injected fetal neural cells. Patients in the sham control arm were exposed to the side effects of this drug and associated risks of infection. They also were exposed to side effects and complications from intravenous antibiotics. Finally, they received radiation from positron emission tomography scans to measure trial outcomes.

The critical ethical commentary on this trial argued that the risks to those receiving the sham intervention were either inherently unethical or too great to be justified by the potential scientific benefit from conducting the research. Certainly, use of the sham intervention presented a heavy burden of proof. The burden was lowered somewhat, however, in the companion trial, which reduced the risks of the sham control by using local anesthesia and omitting immunosuppressive treatment [38]. Others argued that the sham-controlled trials were justified [31,39].

It is notable that the critics made sweeping categorical claims that sham surgery is necessarily or presumptively unethical, based on ethical analysis of one study of sham-controlled fetal tissue transplantation. Comparison with the sham controls used in the less risky alternative trial, the much lower-risk trial of internal mammary artery ligation, and the report of a pilot study of sham-controlled arthroscopic surgery [40] might have suggested that the ethical justifiability of sham surgery depends on the risk-benefit ratios presented by different trials. It is useful to examine in detail a more recent case, which exposed patients to sham surgery with considerably less risk than in the fetal tissue transplantation trials.

Arthroscopic surgery

A randomized placebo-controlled clinical trial of arthroscopic surgery for osteoarthritis of the knee evaluated two surgical procedures in comparison with a sham operation [8]. The study included 180 patients with knee arthritis who reported at least moderate knee pain despite maximal medical treatment for at least 6 months. They were randomized to three study arms: (1) arthroscopic debridement, (2) arthroscopic lavage, or (3) a sham operation. The primary outcome measure was knee pain 2 years after surgery. The relatively minor risks to those receiving the sham operation derived from side effects of anesthesia involving an intravenous tranquilizer and opioid drug, and from discomfort and potential complications associated with three 1-cm skin incisions to the knee. The study report noted two minor postoperative complications among research participants, neither of whom received the sham intervention (N. Wray, personal communication, 2002).

To promote informed consent, the research participants were required to write in their medical charts the following statement: "On entering this study, I realize that I may receive only placebo surgery. I further realize that this means that I will not have surgery on my knee joint. This placebo surgery will not benefit my knee arthritis" [8]. Of those patients who were eligible and invited to participate in the study, 44% declined to do so.

Ethical analysis

The ethical analysis of sham surgery presented here, focusing primarily on the case of arthroscopic surgery, examines five key ethical questions [41]:

1. Did the research question have scientific and clinical value?
2. Was the use of sham surgery as a control intervention methodologically necessary or desirable to achieve valid results?
3. Were the risks minimized for subjects randomized to sham surgery?
4. Were the risks of the sham surgery that were not balanced by the prospect of medical benefits within a reasonable threshold of acceptable research risk?
5. Were the risks of the sham intervention justified by the potential value of the scientific knowledge to be gained from the research?

Scientific and clinical value

Arthroscopic surgery for arthritis of the knee is a common procedure, which had been introduced into clinical practice without rigorous evaluation of its efficacy. Moseley and coworkers [8] estimated that it has been performed 650,000 times per year in the United States, at an approximate cost of $5000 per procedure. In open studies, about one half of patients reported relief of pain, although the physiologic basis for pain relief is unclear. A RCT evaluating rigorously the efficacy of a common and expensive surgical procedure would certainly make a valuable contribution to scientific knowledge and clinical practice.

Methodologic rationale for sham control

The primary outcome that this trial was designed to measure was relief of pain—an inherently subjective phenomenon. Is a sham-controlled trial methodologically necessary to determine whether arthroscopic surgery is effective in relieving pain caused by osteoarthritis of the knee? To answer this question depends on comparing a sham-controlled trial design with the most reasonable alternative study design of a randomized trial of arthroscopic surgery versus standard medical treatment. In the alternative trial, patients could not be blind to treatment assignment. The lack of masked treatment could produce biased assessments of knee pain and function. Patients might be inclined to report that they felt better because they knew that they had received surgery. Although outcome raters initially could be blind to which intervention trial participants received, their remaining blind would depend on patients not openly or suggestively communicating whether or not they received surgery. A recently reported study of surgery versus splinting for carpal tunnel syndrome revealed that, even though patients were encouraged not to disclose their treatment to outcome raters, "many patients inadvertently mentioned their treatment" [42].

Weijer [35], in a commentary on the ethics of the fetal tissue transplantation trial, discounted the importance of blind conditions in a trial of surgery versus medical treatment by noting that unblinded but valid randomized trials have been used to evaluate chemotherapy versus radiation for the treatment of cancer. The comparison, however, is not apt; these cancer trials measure objective outcomes, such as mortality, tumor shrinkage, and recurrence of disease, which are not subject to the biases associated with subjective ratings [43].

Moreover, trials of surgery versus medical treatment do not control for the potential placebo effects of surgery. Reduced pain and improved knee function may result from the psychologic influence of receiving an invasive procedure and believing or hoping that it works, rather than from any specific effects of debridement or lavage. Is the placebo effect of surgery real? Beecher [1] certainly was overconfident in concluding that "a placebo effect has been demonstrated for surgery." The results of the sham-controlled internal mammary artery trials, which prompted this conclusion, demonstrated dramatic evidence of patient improvement following the sham operation. Strictly speaking, they did not show that the observed improvement was caused by the sham surgery. Although perhaps unlikely, the observed improvement might have reflected spontaneous remission or symptomatic fluctuation, the therapeutic benefit of close clinical attention, or biased responses of patients. Just as observed responses following drug administration must be distinguished from true drug effects, so must an observed response to placebo be distinguished from a true placebo effect that can be attributed to the placebo intervention [44]. Systematic scientific study of the placebo effect in surgery, using a three-arm randomized trial of a real surgery, a sham control, and a no-treatment group, has yet to be conducted.

A recent meta-analysis encompassing a wide range of randomized clinical trials that included both placebo and no-treatment arms called into question the reality of the placebo effect [45]. This study, however, did not include any sham-controlled trials of surgery. Furthermore, pain was the one outcome variable in the meta-analysis most suggestive of a true placebo effect. Although sufficient evidence is lacking to conclude that surgery produces a genuine placebo effect, the potential for sham surgery to produce therapeutic benefit certainly cannot be ruled out. Indeed, there is reason to think, supported by some suggestive evidence, that sham surgery may produce pronounced placebo effects [46–48].

The potential for bias from an unblinded trial of surgery versus medical treatment, coupled with the potential for surgery to produce powerful placebo effects, make it doubtful that a rigorous trial of surgery can be conducted without a sham surgery control when the primary outcome is pain, patient-reported improvement, or quality of life.

Risk-benefit assessment

A basic ethical requirement of clinical research is to minimize risks [26]. This obviously does not mean that risks can be reduced to zero, or that risks must be "minimal." Macklin [32] categorically rejected sham surgery because it fails to satisfy this requirement of minimizing risks: "It is undeniable that performing surgery in research subjects that has no potential therapeutic benefit fails to minimize the risks of harm." The reason for this sweeping claim is that the surgery under investigation could always be evaluated in a study design that poses less risk because it does not involve sham surgery, as in a comparison with standard medical therapy or no treatment. The logic of Macklin's [32] argument, directed at the sham-controlled trial of fetal tissue transplantation, also rules out low-risk sham surgery, exemplified by the arthroscopic surgery trial. This stance, however, rests on a faulty understanding of the requirement of minimizing risks. Risks of research interventions should be minimized consistent with answering valuable scientific questions by rigorous methods. If a less risky alternative study design is not methodologically equipped to answer the question whether a given surgery works, then it is not mandated by the ethical requirement of minimizing risks. Risks are minimized when there is no practicable alternative method of validly testing study hypotheses that poses lower risks. The sham-controlled arthroscopic surgery trial satisfied this requirement. Specifically, this study reduced risks to those receiving the sham operation by using the combination of a sedative and narcotic drug for anesthesia, as an alternative to the standard deep general anesthesia with endotracheal intubation, which was administered to those who received arthroscopic surgery [8]. Nevertheless, the determination that a sham-controlled surgery trial has minimized risks does not imply that the risks of the sham operation are justified.

The question remains whether the level of risk for the sham arthroscopic surgery was excessive or intolerable. The risks from the anesthesia and skin incisions were not high, and certainly were considerably less than in the sham controls for the fetal tissue transplantation trials. The risks were more than minimal, however, which is defined in the United States federal regulations as "the probability and magnitude of harm or discomfort anticipated in the research are not greater in and of themselves than those ordinarily encountered in daily life or during the performance of routine physical or psychological examinations or tests" [49]. These risks, however, seem comparable with, or at least not markedly greater than, the risks of other generally accepted research procedures used in studies that offer no prospect of benefit to subjects, such as muscle biopsies, bronchoscopies, and phase I testing of drugs in healthy volunteers.

The ultimate question of risk-benefit assessment is whether the risks of sham arthroscopic surgery were justified by the anticipated scientific value of the study. There are no objective tools for measuring research risk-benefit ratios. I contend that the moderate risks of the methodologically indicated sham procedure were justifiable to answer the clinically important question of whether arthroscopic surgery is effective to treat pain associated with arthritis of the knee. This is a matter of judgment, about which reasonable people may differ.

Consequences of not performing sham-controlled trials

The ethical analysis presented here has been devoted to the question whether it ever can be ethical to use sham surgery in a clinical trial. Yet, the methodologic rationale and risk-benefit assessment for using sham surgery in the arthroscopic surgery trial suggest the opposite question. Can it be ethical not to use sham surgery to evaluate rigorously a surgical procedure under the following conditions: when methodologic reasons indicate that a sham surgery control is needed to demonstrate efficacy, and the risks of the sham procedure are not excessive and justified by the value of the knowledge to be gained from the study?

Arthroscopic surgery has been widely used to relieve pain from arthritis of the knee despite lacking rigorous evaluation. The recent sham-controlled trial showed that two methods of surgery were no better than a sham operation [8]. It follows that many patients have been exposed to risks for a nonbeneficial treatment, and that those who have paid for these procedures have been wasting money.

Informed consent

As indicated in discussing the problems with the therapeutic orientation to clinical research, the distinction between clinical research and clinical care has important implications for informed consent. At the very least, patients exposed to surgical investigation that is the object of study should be informed that they are participating in research. Innovative practice that involves research without so informing patients violates this principle. Furthermore, to avoid the therapeutic misconception, informed consent to research participation should clarify the differences between being in research and receiving standard therapy. Several studies indicate that a sizeable proportion of participants in RCTs fail to understand randomization [19,50,51]. Despite being informed that the treatment they will receive in the trial is determined by chance, many participants report the belief that their treatment is selected according to a judgment of what is medically best for them. It is not surprising that this therapeutic misconception occurs, because randomization is foreign to the ethos of clinical care. In surgical trials that compare a surgical procedure with a less invasive medical procedure or pharmacologic therapy understanding randomization is especially important. Subjects need to comprehend that by agreeing to participate in the trial they are forgoing the opportunity for them or their physician to choose between these very different forms of treatment. A recent review of research on interventions aimed at improving the informed consent of research participants found that the most effective method of enhancing understanding is extended discussion regarding the research protocol by a member of the study team or a neutral educator [52].

Sham surgery trials raise distinctive issues of informed consent, because of the fact that the surgeon is not blind to whether the patient-subject is receiving a real or sham procedure. To keep patients from knowing what intervention they received, surgical investigators may need to use misleading or deceptive tactics to induce belief among those randomized to the sham operation that they are in fact receiving a real surgery [32,53]. The report of the arthroscopic surgery study described the sham operation as follows: "The surgeon asked for all the instruments and manipulated the knee as if arthroscopy was being performed. Saline was splashed to simulate the sounds of lavage" [8]. Given that the subjects were likely to be asleep before the sham operation was performed, one might argue that these misleading tactics were harmless. Local anesthesia, however, was used in the internal mammary artery ligation trial and one of the trials of fetal tissue transplantation. For cases in which patients are not put to sleep before the sham operation, misleading tactics pose genuine ethical qualms.

The key ethical issue is whether the deception is wrongful. Can it be ethical for investigators deliberately to mislead trial participants about the nature of the treatment they are receiving? The answer depends critically on whether subjects were informed about the use of such misleading tactics before agreeing to enroll in the trial. If they were informed that the surgeon investigator would be making efforts to mimic the real surgery, then subjects were not being wrongfully deceived [54]. Their signing the consent document signified prospective authorization for the misleading tactics. The arthroscopic surgery trial might be faulted for not making this clear in the informed consent process (N. Wray, personal communication, 2002), but the omission is discounted by the expectation that patients would be asleep at the time the sham operation was performed. Moreover, to promote understanding and appreciation of the use of a sham surgery control, the informed consent process for this trial adopted the novel and exemplary safeguard of requiring participants to write in their own hand that they realized the chance that they might receive a placebo surgery.

Summary

Higher standards of evidence for surgical procedures are likely to be demanded in the future by health insurance providers [55]. Consequently, more formal and rigorous surgical research, including RCTs, will become more prevalent. Facing the ethical challenges of surgical research requires understanding of the ethically significant differences between surgical practice and research and the ways in which the ethical standards appropriate for the design and conduct of clinical research differ from the ethics of clinical care.

References

[1] Beecher HK. Surgery as placebo. JAMA 1961;176: 88–93.
[2] Horton R. Surgical research or comic opera: questions but few answers. Lancet 1996;347:984.
[3] McCulloch P, Taylor I, Sasako M, et al. Randomized trials in surgery: problems and possible solutions. BMJ 2002;394:1448–51.
[4] Porter R. The greatest benefit to mankind. New York: WW Norton; 1998.
[5] Cobb LA, Thomas GI, Dillard DH, et al. An evaluation of internal-mammary artery ligation by a double-blind technique. N Engl J Med 1959;260:1115–8.
[6] Dimond EG, Kittle CG, Crockett JE. Comparison of internal mammary artery ligation and sham operation for angina pectoris. Am J Cardiol 1960;5:484–6.
[7] Deyo RA, Patrick DL. Hope or hype. New York: AMACOM Books; 2005.
[8] Moseley JB, O'Malley K, Petersen NJ, et al. A controlled trial of arthroscopic surgery for osteoarthritis of the knee. N Engl J Med 2002;347:81–8.
[9] van Staaij BK, van den Akker EH, Rovers MM, et al. Effectiveness of adenotonsillectomy in children with mild symptoms of throat infection or adenotonsillar hypertrophy: open randomized trial. BMJ 2004;329:651.
[10] Stirrat GM. Ethics and evidence based surgery. J Med Ethics 2004;30:160–5.
[11] Cassell J. Expected miracles: surgeons at work. Philadelphia: Temple University Press; 1991.
[12] McLeod RS. Issues in surgical randomized controlled trials. World J Surg 1999;23:1210–4.
[13] Reitsma AM, Moreno JD. Surgical research: an elusive entity. Am J Bioeth 2003;3:49–50.
[14] National Commission for the Protection of Human Subjects of Biomedical and Behavioral Research. The Belmont Report. Washington: US Government Printing Office; 1979.
[15] Margo CE. When is surgery research? Towards an operational definition of human research. J Med Ethics 2001;27:40–3.
[16] Reitsma AM, Moreno JD. Ethical regulations for innovative surgery: the last frontier? J Am Coll Surg 2002;194:792–801.
[17] Miller FG, Rosenstein DL. The therapeutic orientation to clinical trials. N Engl J Med 2003;348:1383–6.
[18] Choosing a clinical trial. M.D. Anderson Cancer Center. www.mdanderson.org. Accessed March 14, 2003.
[19] Appelbaum PS, Roth LH, Lidz CW, et al. False hopes and best data: consent to research and the therapeutic misconception. Hastings Cent Rep 1987;17: 20–4.
[20] World Medical Association. Declaration of Helsinki: ethical principles for medical research involving human subjects. JAMA 2000;284:3043–5.
[21] Freedman B. Equipoise and the ethics of clinical research. N Engl J Med 1987;317:141–5.
[22] Freedman B, Glass KC, Weijer C. Placebo orthodoxy in clinical research. II: Ethical, legal and regulatory myths. J Law Med Ethics 1996;24:252–9.
[23] Miller FG, Brody H. A critique of clinical equipoise: therapeutic misconception in the ethics of clinical trials. Hastings Cent Rep 2003;33:19–28.
[24] Gifford F. The conflict between randomized clinical trials and the therapeutic obligation. J Med Philos 1986;11:347–66.
[25] Miller FG, Rosenstein DL, DeRenzo EG. Professional integrity in clinical research. JAMA 1998;280: 1449–54.
[26] Emanuel EJ, Wendler D, Grady C. What makes research ethical? JAMA 2000;283:2701–11.
[27] Miller FG. Sham surgery: an ethical analysis. Am J Bioeth 2003;3:41–8.
[28] Frader JE, Caniano DA. Research and innovation in surgery. In: McCullough LB, Jones JW, Brody BA, editors. Surgical ethics. New York: Oxford University Press; 1998. p. 216–41.
[29] Clark PA. Placebo surgery for Parkinson's diseases: do the benefits outweigh the risks? J Law Med Ethics 2002;30:58–68.
[30] London AJ, Kadane JB. Placebos that harm: sham surgery controls in clinical trials. Stat Methods Med Res 2002;11:413–27.
[31] Freeman TB, Vawter DE, Leaverton PE, et al. Use of placebo surgery in controlled trials of a cellular-based therapy for Parkinson's disease. N Engl J Med 1999; 341:988–91.
[32] Macklin R. The ethical problem with sham surgery in clinical research. N Engl J Med 1999;341:992–6.
[33] Dekkers W, Boer GB. Sham neurosurgery in patients with Parkinson's disease: is it morally acceptable? J Med Ethics 2001;27:151–6.
[34] Gillett GR. Unnecessary holes in the head. IRB 2001; 23:1–6.
[35] Weijer C. I need a placebo like I need a hole in the head. J Law Med Ethics 2002;30:69–72.
[36] Albin RL. Sham surgery controls: intracerebral grafting of fetal tissue for Parkinson's disease and proposed criteria for use of sham surgery controls. J Med Ethics 2002;28:322–5.
[37] Advisory Committee on Human Radiation Experiments. Final report. Washington: US Government Printing Office; 1995.
[38] Freed CR, Greene PE, Breeze RE, et al. Transplantation of embryonic dopamine neurons for severe Parkinson's disease. N Engl J Med 2001;344:710–9.
[39] Fletcher JC. Sham neurosurgery in Parkinson's disease: ethical at the time. Am J Bioeth 2003;3:54–6.
[40] Moseley JB, Wray NP, Kuykendall D, et al. Arthro-

scopic treatment of osteoarthritis of the knee: a prospective, randomized, placebo-controlled trial. Results of a pilot study. Am J Sports Med 1996;24:28–34.
[41] Horng S, Miller FG. Is placebo surgery ethical? N Engl J Med 2002;347:137–9.
[42] Gerritsen AAM, de Vet HCW, Scholten BJPM, et al. Splinting vs surgery in the treatment of carpal tunnel syndrome. JAMA 2002;288:1245–51.
[43] Lasagna L. The controlled clinical trial: theory and practice. J Chronic Dis 1955;1:353–67.
[44] Ernst E, Resch KL. Concept of true and perceived placebo effects. BMJ 1995;311:551–3.
[45] Hrobjartsson A, Gotzsche PC. Is the placebo powerless? N Engl J Med 2001;344:1594–602.
[46] Johnson AG. Surgery as a placebo. Lancet 1994;344:1140–2.
[47] Kaptchuk TJ, Goldman P, Stone DA, et al. Do medical devices have enhanced placebo effects? J Clin Epidemiol 2000;53:786–92.
[48] Moerman DE, Jonas WB. Deconstructing the placebo effect and finding the meaning response. Ann Intern Med 2002;136:471–6.
[49] Department of Health and Human Services. Protection of human subjects. 45 CFR §46 (1991).
[50] Criscione LG, Sugarman J, Sanders L, et al. Informed consent in a clinical trial of a novel treatment for rheumatoid arthritis. Arthritis Rheum 2003;49:361–7.
[51] Kodish E, Eder M, Noll RB, et al. Communication of randomization in childhood leukemia trials. JAMA 2004;291:470–5.
[52] Flory J, Emanuel E. Interventions to improve research participants' understanding in informed consent for research: a systematic review. JAMA 2004;292:1593–601.
[53] Miller FG, Kaptchuk TJ. Sham procedures and the ethics of clinical trials. J R Soc Med 2004;97:576–8.
[54] Wendler D, Miller FG. Deception in the pursuit of science. Arch Intern Med 2004;164:597–600.
[55] Ramsey SD, Sullivan SD. Evidence, economics, and emphysema: Medicare's long journey with lung volume reduction surgery. Health Aff (Millwood) 2005;24:55–65.

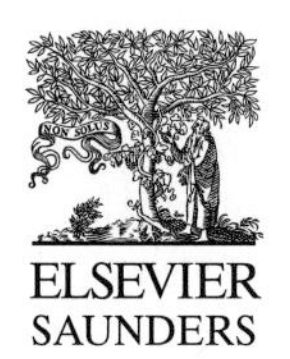
ELSEVIER
SAUNDERS

Thorac Surg Clin 15 (2005) 555 – 563

THORACIC
SURGERY
CLINICS

Surgically Implanted Devices: Ethical Challenges in a Very Different Kind of Research

E. Haavi Morreim, PhD

College of Medicine, University of Tennessee Health Science Center, 956 Court, Suite B328, Memphis, TN 38163, USA

In recent years clinical medical research has come under increasing public scrutiny. Much of that attention has focused on such issues as whether this or that study has been tainted by conflicts of interest, whether drugs are sometimes approved with too little long-term follow-up, and whether study designs have adequately observed the principles of ethically and scientifically credible research. For the most part, the ethics and regulations of clinical research are based on a drug model, with relatively little attention to devices. Although research on surgically implanted devices can raise issues familiar from drug studies, this article suggests they can also raise special challenges.

Readers of *Thoracic Surgery Clinics* are considerably more familiar with device trials than most observers of medical research. Nonetheless, it is useful to highlight some of the major differences between drug and device trials. This article suggests some ways in which device trials can raise distinctive ethical issues. Throughout the AbioCor artificial heart trial is used as an example. Although this particular trial should not be deemed typical of surgically implanted device studies, it can highlight some particularly significant methodologic and ethical features.

During the AbioCor trial, the author served as chair of the Independent Patient Advocacy Council (IPAC), whose patient advocate members provided assistance to patients and families participating in the trial. Although initiated by ABIOMED, the IPAC was independent of the corporation. It was funded by a lump sum, irrevocable trust; the group chose its own members other than the first few, and defined its own mission and activities.

E-mail address: hmorreim@utmem.edu

The AbioCor study

The AbioCor, manufactured by ABIOMED (Danvers, Massachusetts), a small Massachusetts corporation, is a totally implantable biventricular replacement device. It has four implanted components [1–4]. The thoracic unit, weighing about 2 lb, consists of right and left ventricles, valves, and a motor-driven hydraulic pumping system. It is anastomosed to the patient's native atria. The controller monitors the heart's function, controlling heart rate and motor speed, which in turn determines the pressure with which blood is forced out of either ventricle. An internal lithium battery can last up to half an hour, and is recharged through the transcutaneous energy transmission system. In the transcutaneous energy transmission system, internal and external coils transmit energy and data across the skin, requiring no percutaneous tubes or wires to invite infection. The external transcutaneous energy transmission is held in place with a soft cloth harness. Other external components include a console that provides a broader system of controls and monitoring, and which can transmit power to recharge the internal battery. Alternatively, a patient-carried electronics system includes battery packs that permit the patient to be completely free of fixed power sources for up to 4 hours at a time. The AbioCor's goal is to promote quality and duration of life (Fig. 1) [5].

The initial feasibility study, as approved by the Food and Drug Administration (FDA), specified that there would be 15 patients in irreversible biventricular failure who are on maximal medical support, ineligible for cardiac transplantation, and within 30 days of death. According to ABIOMED, the potential

1547-4127/05/$ – see front matter
doi:10.1016/j.thorsurg.2005.06.009

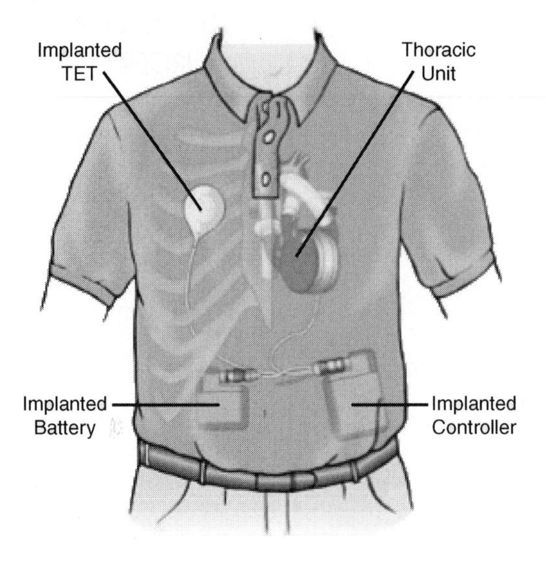

Fig. 1. The AbioCor device. (Courtesy of Abiomed, Inc., Danvers, MA; with permission.)

patient population includes persons who are unlikely to benefit from long-term ventricular assist devices, and who may have such conditions as [6]:

Severe right ventricular failure, in addition to severe left ventricular failure
Pulmonary hypertension refractory to pharmacologic management
Significant aortic valve regurgitation
Mechanical valve prosthesis
Intractable life-threatening arrhythmias
Massive acute myocardial infarction with friable tissue
Ventricular septal rupture
Failed heart transplant (rejection) with immunosuppression
Thrombus in the ventricles

On July 2, 2001, the first human implant took place in Louisville, Kentucky. The five other study sites designated for the first 15 patients are Houston, Los Angeles, Philadelphia, Boston, and Tucson. At press time, 14 of the 15 implants have taken place, mostly in Louisville and Houston.

Results have been mixed but fairly encouraging, given the context of first human use of a completely new device. One patient survived nearly a year and a half and was discharged home for 7 months. Eleven others survived from periods of nearly 2 months to over 9 months, and of these, two were able to make various excursions outside the hospital. Two died perioperatively. Two instances of device failure occurred, one of which was anticipated and the other of which, although unexpected, was analyzed and addressed to avoid future occurrences [7,8]. Significant morbidities were reported, many of them related to the patients' poor state of preoperative health, and some caused by postoperative strokes associated with thromboembolism. Thromboembolic events are being addressed by a modification of the device, by ongoing refinement of the anticoagulation protocols, and by optimizing device and patient management [2–4].

Drug trials versus device trials: standardization versus incremental innovation

With these basic features of the AbioCor study outlined, I now discuss how surgically implanted device trials such as this differ from the routine drug trial. It should be emphasized that this case study is used purely for illustrative purposes, and should not be considered typical of implanted devices. Indeed, it might reasonably be said that there is no such thing as a typical device or device trial. Additionally, the AbioCor trial is actually a feasibility study (essentially the equivalent of a pre–phase I effort), not the more classic phase I, II, or III research. Nevertheless, this case study highlights some important differences that can arise between drug and device trials.

At the outset, drug studies commonly include large numbers of subjects [9]. Drugs often produce only incremental changes, or incremental differences over existing drugs, and usually require large numbers to show statistical significance.

To produce scientifically generalizable results, a study ordinarily must be carefully controlled so that differences in outcomes can be attributed to the intervention being evaluated rather than to happenstance events or to extraneous features, such as personal differences among research subjects. Accordingly, drug studies commonly are hypothesis-driven and use methodologic techniques such as double-blinding, randomization, and placebo-controls.

These controls mean that activities in the typical drug study are highly standardized. The protocol dictates precisely what will happen, when, and how. Subjects are placed in a given arm by randomization, not choice. If the study says they will receive X dose rather than the Y dose they or their physician might prefer, they nonetheless receive X. If the protocol says that certain tests are done on day 5, they are done on day 5, not day 4, not day 6; and it is those tests, not some other tests.

Only limited flexibility is allowed in the typical drug trial (eg, perhaps to allow adjuvant medications for symptom relief). If enrollees or investigators were permitted to use any medications they wished or to vary the trial intervention any way they wanted, the study's results could be completely confounded. The only option if research participation causes undue harm or discomfort is simply to remove that person from the study. Unplanned variation is anathema to the typical drug trial.

Implanted device trials are very different. Standard controls are often either impossible or undesirable. Double-blinding is usually precluded by the surgeon's need to see what he or she is doing, although postoperative evaluations can sometimes be undertaken by blinded, independent observers. Randomization may be unacceptable or unfeasible where prospective enrollees are unwilling to leave to chance the question whether they will receive a major intervention like surgical device implantation. Placebo controls like sham surgery may be ethically acceptable only under very limited conditions [10–13].

Where drug trials usually need to be large, an implanted device trial can be surprisingly small. A device like the AbioCor, used in people who are clearly expected to die very soon, can potentially produce very dramatic results that require far fewer enrolled subjects to demonstrate efficacy [14,15]. At the same time, if in the future some other device or modality seems to produce results similar to the AbioCor in the same population, a considerably larger trial would be required to discern which is superior.

Additionally, most devices have far smaller target populations than the typical drug, with commensurately fewer people eligible to participate in a research trial. Moreover, willingness to participate may be considerably smaller where the requirement is to undergo a surgery and sometimes also to pay for part or all of one's participation in the trial. Because many device manufacturers are small firms, their financial ability to support large trials is sharply limited.

Further compounding these challenges are the learning curves both for the device and for clinicians. Regarding learning curve for the device itself, Ramsey and coworkers [16] note that "[u]nlike the development of pharmaceuticals, device development is often iterative and ongoing. Device modifications are constantly made over time in response to clinical testing and user preferences." Similarly, Witkin [15] observed that "[f]requent innovations in the design and use of medical devices are standard practice in the industry. These are often minor modifications that enhance safety, reliability, patient comfort, or ease of use...."

Consistent with this pattern, the AbioCor underwent a midtrial modification. Following major cerebrovascular accidents in several of the early enrollees, the company first removed, then modified and reintroduced a "cage" or "inflow stent." The stent helps to keep the atrial walls open as blood flow from the atria to the ventricles creates significant negative pressure. The redesigned stent is intended to reduce the potential for thromboembolic events and obstructive inflow limitations.

Surgeons' implantation techniques can travel an even greater learning curve. Partly, this comes from improvements in surgeons' skills as they become more comfortable with implantation procedures. Additionally, those procedures themselves may be refined as the trial goes forward.

Postoperative device and patient management can introduce still more evolution. Some devices, like the AbioCor, are physiologically active after implantation. Rather than being largely inert like the typical orthopedic implant, a device like the AbioCor significantly affects patients' physiologic functioning, both directly by circulating blood and indirectly by enhancing organ function via increased oxygenation and perfusion. In the presence of such physiologic activity, a major objective of such a study usually involves exploring how best to manage the device and patient postoperatively. The AbioCor trial, for instance, witnessed significant changes in anticoagulation protocols over the course of the first dozen patients [2].

This evolutionary factor poses a familiar challenge for any surgical innovation [17,18], not just those associated with implanted device trials. So long as this sort of evolution is under way, it may be counterproductive to try to measure its efficacy or appropriateness too early. If a new approach is tested immediately, before the initial problems have been identified and worked out, then by the time the study is completed, it is almost surely out of date [19,20]. No matter when any such testing begins, however, the evolutionary process is likely to continue. Rarely is there a clear moment at which to say, "Now it is finalized and ready for definitive evaluation." Surgery trials are often ill-suited to the rigorous standardization required for the typical drug trial, because premature or undue standardization could preclude the very improvements that could optimize patient care.

Several conclusions emerge from these observations. First, whereas in a drug trial unplanned variation is often an anathema, such variation is often an important and desirable constituent of a device trial, particularly in the early stages. In such a setting there are few if any rigid scientific "protocols." At most there are tentative rules of thumb that can guide physicians until and unless there is reason to do something else. But if there is any reason to ignore such an informal protocol, then it is ignored. Any anticoagulation protocol in the AbioCor trial, for instance, was immediately suspended or modified if a patient developed a bleeding episode. Other issues, such as nutrition, rehabilitation, infections, and so forth, were addressed similarly. In sum, conduct that might in a drug trial represent an unwanted glitch at best, or even scientific misconduct, can signify learning and productivity in an implanted device trial.

Second, unlike classic drug research, this sort of study truly does aim at the best personal interests of each enrolled subject. The typical drug trial must not claim to promote any particular individual's best interest because, per the requisites of scientific rigor, what happens to any individual is determined not by what might best meet his or her personal needs and desires, but what the protocol says must happen. They are assigned to a specific treatment arm (or to placebo) by randomization, and they receive test X on day 5 and test Y on day 10 because this is how scientifically generalizable results are reached. Individuals may benefit, but that is by fortunate happenstance, not by design.

In a study like the AbioCor, most of the effort directly aims to maximize each recipient's chances at surviving and enjoying the best possible quality of life. The better each individual does, the better the trial does, unlike the drug study in which the manufacturers must fervently hope that not everyone does equally well, and that those who receive the new drug fare distinctly better than those who receive placebo or existing drugs.

Finally, what happens during a device trial, particularly during a device's earliest human trials, is not actually "research" in any standard sense. It is inquiry, innovation, problem-solving, even experimentation. But it is not "research" as defined by federal regulations: "Research means a systematic investigation, including research development, testing, and evaluation, designed to develop or contribute to generalizable knowledge" [21,22]. Where the investigator simply tries one thing and then another, as idiosyncratically as necessary, to see what works for a particular patient, the result is not scientific generalizability. The investigator may glean some useful lessons and insights that might be tried for the next patient, but ultimately the next person is another experiment with an "n" of one. At the same time, other investigators at the trial's other sites may try a very different approach to a similar problem, further enhancing the chance of learning from such early experiences. Eventually these insights may make it possible to craft a more traditional kind of bona fide research trial, although even then, as a device trial it is still importantly different from familiar drug trials.

Ethical challenges specific to device trials

Device trials like the AbioCor study, which features patients facing the end of life, a very new implanted device with substantial uncertainties, and a significant need for as-you-go innovation, raise a number of interesting issues.

Innovation and collaboration

Trials like this require abundant innovation. In some instances the questions to be answered are not clear until experience starkly presents them. The clinical team must then resolve, largely through an iterative, trial and error process, such questions as what is the best surgical implantation procedure, optimal anticoagulation, optimal rates of flow, and other matters. This is innovation, but not research.

Such flexibility, however, does not exempt the investigators from the responsibility to proceed with great care. They need to base their innovations on sound clinical judgment and the broadest possible information base. Throughout the AbioCor study, the surgeons and other collaborating physicians at the study's six sites periodically gathered together with ABIOMED's corporate executives and with a number of independent surgeons and physicians to review what successes and problems had arisen to date, what approach the teams at each site had taken to resolve those problems and why, and what outcomes had resulted. The group then discussed how best to proceed, whether current strategies seemed to be working, or whether they should be modified, and why and how. In some instances a consensus developed around a single approach that all sites would implement for the foreseeable future (unless it did not seem appropriate for a particular patient.) In other instances the group identified two or more approaches, allowing each site its option of preference. Updated results were shared at subsequent meetings as a foundation for whatever further evolution might be warranted.

This sort of ongoing, systematic communication and collaboration is both medically and ethically desirable. Unfortunately, it is more the exception than the rule, even in major device trials. Although a diversity of approaches can be highly desirable, and sometimes can more quickly lead to workable solutions for difficult problems, it makes little sense for each study site to reinvent the wheel, or to fail to learn from each other's successes and misadventures.

Patient selection

As with other trials of potentially life-saving but novel medical interventions, such as new chemotherapy agents for cancer, the FDA specified that the first people to receive the AbioCor must be very near the end of life and lacking any medical or surgical alternatives [23]. Because the device was highly experimental, it was deemed inappropriate to enroll people who still have a reasonable life expectancy or viable medical alternatives.

Such a limitation, however, still left an important choice. Many of the people who qualified for this trial had experienced prolonged, progressive heart failure. Others were previously healthy victims of a sudden, massive myocardial infarction from which recovery is highly unlikely. From a purely medical standpoint the latter group is often preferable candidates, because those patients ordinarily have little or none of the organ damage that commonly accompanies end-stage heart failure. Additionally, some of those individuals might value the chance to speak with their loved ones, to set their affairs in order, or to undertake some of the other end-of-life tasks that are otherwise precluded when death comes suddenly and unexpectedly.

Unfortunately, acute myocardial infarction patients are often heavily sedated and unable to participate in a decision about whether to enroll in a highly experimental research trial, and in most cases little evidence exists about what they would say if competent. Relatively few of these people have had serious prior conversations about high-risk research participation, or even about the merits of aggressive end-of-life care.

This dearth of patient input poses a serious problem. Under more routine circumstances it is standard for a person's next of kin to make decisions on that person's behalf. There are limits, however, on the kinds of decisions that any person can make on behalf of another; on what parents can choose for their children, even from altruistic motives; or what an adult daughter could choose on behalf of her father with Alzheimer's disease.

If an Alzheimer patient has expressed, while competent, an explicit wish to participate in research, then enrolling him or her may be acceptable. Absent any indication whether this patient wants to participate in research, however, there are strong ethical limits on the risk to which such a person should be subjected in the name of gathering research information. Children provide a useful illustration. When there is no chance that they can personally benefit from the proposed research, children can be exposed only to minimal risk (the kinds of risk they face every day as part of life) or to a minor increase over minimal risk. If there is a chance of benefit from the research, then somewhat greater risks can be accepted, but they must be proportional to the potential for benefit.

An adult who is currently incompetent and whose preferences about such a project are completely unknown does not have the same legal status as a child, yet ethically a comparable norm may apply. It is difficult to argue that participation in such a high-risk study, at such an early stage, is a benefit, given the great uncertainties and lack of track record at that juncture. It is entirely possible, at that initial stage in the study, that such a device might only prolong suffering and delay dying. Indeed, it is common for early trials of implanted devices to experience very high rates of failure [24]. Equally important, when the prospective enrollee has been unable to hear about the project's potential risks and benefits, he or she also has had no opportunity to present any considered values about quality of life and end of life, to provide concrete indications of the conditions under which he or she wants to cease participation in the trial and thereby, in this setting, to die.

Accordingly, although the FDA would have permitted surrogate enrollment in the trial, ABIOMED implemented an informal policy requiring that the first people to enroll in the AbioCor study should be competent to provide informed consent: to hear available information regarding the device, the study, the uncertainties, and the potential risks and benefits, and to make their own decision in light of their own values. For similar reasons, the institutional review board (IRB) at one of the six trial-sites imposed its own local restriction limiting the trial to competent patients only.

Only after the first 14 patients had been enrolled did the company determine that the uncertainties had been sufficiently reduced to permit surrogate decision making to enroll someone in the trial (although the IRB restriction at the one site noted previously maintained its exclusion on surrogate enrollment). Even so, it is still important for the surgeon to discern from families, up front, whether there is credible reason to believe that this person would agree that entering the trial is desirable.

Best interests and the therapeutic misconception

Scientific research focuses on producing generalizable knowledge. The requisite standardization of interventions and measurements means that most of what happens to an enrollee is chosen, not for their benefit, but to promote the research goals. In contrast, although a feasibility study, such as the AbioCor trial, does evaluate the device, what actually happens to any implant recipient is largely determined by what is best for that individual person. The better each patient does, the better do the trial and the device.

As a result, such trials are much less subject to a serious problem in most clinical trials, namely the "therapeutic misconception." The therapeutic misconception (TM) refers to the mistaken belief held by many research subjects that virtually everything that happens in a research trial is tailored to their personal benefit. Notwithstanding lengthy explanations of randomization, double-blinding, placebo controls and the like, many subjects cling to the belief that their doctor will personally choose whatever interventions are individually best for them [25,26]. The TM represents a problem, because it may be illusory to suppose that one has truly gotten an informed consent when the enrolled subjects are so profoundly mistaken about the nature and purpose of the research enterprise.

In the AbioCor study and in similar early device trials, this TM worry is largely moot. The enrollee is quite right to believe that physicians will do their utmost to promote his or her personal benefit. A major problem of informed consent is largely bypassed.

There is, however, a caveat. It is quite possible that investigators in such a study may at least occasionally want to undertake some intervention, such as a diagnostic test, whose purpose may be purely to learn more about device function or some other investigational goal. Where a proposed intervention is not for this particular patient's benefit, and is unlikely to enhance his or her welfare or improve medical management, a special informed consent issue arises.

If such an intervention is desired, the request should be explained to the patient or surrogate, describing what the investigators would like to do and why, emphasizing that it is not for the patient's benefit and that he or she has the right to refuse with no compromise in the care that will otherwise be provided.

The investigators should not evade such special informed consent conversations in the mistaken belief that the patient somehow agreed to this sort of thing up front in the original consent form. Because early device trials feature incremental iterations of change, the extra interventions that investigators might eventually want to undertake are virtually impossible to anticipate and explicitly include in the consent form. At most the form might say, "There may be some tests or other interventions we will want to undertake, solely to learn more about the device." Such a notation, however, is not specific enough to count in a bona fide informed consent. Unless the intervention was explicitly identified at the outset, along with its known risks and benefits, a generic "maybe we will want to do other things as yet unspecified" cannot suffice.

It is unclear how formal such a special consent must be. Ethically, it may be acceptable to conduct an informal conversation with appropriate documentation in the patient's medical record. If the nonbeneficial intervention poses any significant risk or discomfort for the patient, however, the investigator is well-advised to work with the local IRB. This is the body that must officially evaluate and approve human research, that provided the initial permission for the study to go forward at that given site, and that is charged with ongoing monitoring of the research projects it has approved. In this sort of instance, the IRB is responsible for ensuring that the risk-benefit balance is acceptable and that the consent process is adequate. Additionally, a failure to work through the IRB could precipitate regulatory repercussions.

If one form of the TM is avoided, another is not. Although patients are correct to think that physicians are generally pursuing their best interests in this sort of device study, they may be wrongly tempted to assume that the device itself is a benefit. In early trials of a major device, the uncertainties are enormous and failure is more the norm than success. Early patients receiving left ventricular assist devices often died [24]. Hemodialysis did not succeed until the seventeenth patient; mitral commissurotomy did not succeed until the fifth patient, and had only 5 successes among first 15; coronary artery bypass graft surgery succeeded for the first patient but then failed for next four. Similar stories can be told regarding cardiac valve replacement, pacemakers, intra-aortic balloon pumps, arterial grafts, and organ transplants [27].

Even so, the first recipients may be tempted to regard this device as their salvation. Because they are close to death, the device is probably their only hope for survival. It does not follow, however, that an only hope is a good or well-founded hope. Moreover, devices and surgical procedures in themselves may have a strong placebo effect, exacerbating this variant of the TM [28].

Probably the best way to address this form of therapeutic misconception is with careful conversations that go beyond the usual informed consent information, as discussed in the next section.

Additional informed consent challenges

Early trials of high-risk implantable devices commonly feature major uncertainties. Although trial sponsors must identify the risks as best they can, and although animal studies can reduce uncertainties up to a point, some eventualities cannot be anticipated. Hence, the initial informed consent document is at best an educated guesstimate of what might befall the first enrollees.

Nevertheless, the informed consent process can be significantly enhanced for later enrollees. Such trials are usually unblinded and relatively small, and as the study progresses, accumulated experience and refinements can substantially reduce uncertainties and clarify the risks. Accordingly, it may sometimes be desirable to revise the consent form partway through such a trial, once sufficient data have accumulated to clarify the risks while protecting prior patients' privacy.

Such revisions are not required. *Goodman v United States* [29] concerned a National Institutes of Health trial for cancer with metastases to liver, in which isolated liver perfusion provided direct injection of drug into the liver. When JoAnn Goodman died after developing liver toxicity from the melphalan and veno-occlusive disease, her husband sued, arguing that National Institutes of Health physicians failed to warn his wife of the foreseeable risks involved in the surgery and thereby failed to obtain legally effective informed consent.

The Ninth Circuit Court of Appeal held that the investigators were not required to inform prospective enrollees about prior patients' courses [29].

> As the district court recognized, "there is no legal requirement that the consent form developed for [the isolated liver perfusion] study must be amended as each group of patients proceeds through the study." To hold that the signed consent form was inadequate would require the National Institutes of Health to update its already detailed consent form every time a patient experiences any sort of complication from an experimental procedure. The National Institutes of Health was not required to update the consent form under these circumstances. The consent form and procedures were medically reasonable and legally adequate.

Although not mandatory, an updated consent form summarizing prior patients' experience can be helpful to give otherwise hypothetical risks a proper tone of reality. During the AbioCor trial, a temporary hiatus after the seventh patient provided such an opportunity. The updated consent form indicated that several patients had experienced a stroke, that some patients had improved enough to become ambulatory, and several other relevant events. The modified version was cleared with the FDA and disseminated to the trial sites. Local IRBs then inserted whatever further modifications they deemed appropriate.

Withdrawing from an implanted device trial

A standard feature of clinical research is the subjects' right to withdraw from the project without prejudicing their ordinary medical care. Prospective subjects are also promised that as the trial progresses, they will be informed of any major developments that might affect their willingness to continue in the study. Presentation of such information usually requires "reconsenting" the subject.

Clearly, a major distinction between implanted device trials and most other clinical studies is that it is often impossible for an enrollee to withdraw once the device has been implanted; obviously true for an artificial heart, but also true for many other devices that cannot be explanted without doing grave harm to the patient. The "reconsenting" idea seems hollow at best.

This does not, however, preclude a patient from deciding that he or she does not wish to contribute further to the data-gathering. If he or she is doing well with an AbioCor, perhaps discharged home, he or she can decline to return for clinical follow-up visits, or can stipulate that new information about his or her condition will no longer be added to the database. More importantly, if a patient is doing poorly and wishes to withdraw entirely, and thereby to die, he or she is also entitled to do so.

In a study like the AbioCor, this possibility requires advance planning. Because the initial patients in this trial were competent to make their own decisions, and because these mortally ill patients could end up in a state they might consider worse than death, an important part of the informed consent process involved careful conversations about personal values regarding quality of life and end of life. The decision when to stop can be at least as important as the decision whether to begin, and it was important to elicit these patients' views at a time when they were still capable of reflection.

Although patients' values differed, many believed that if they became permanently incapable of communicating or participating in relationships with their families, this would be the threshold beyond which further life would not be worthwhile. As the trial progressed and several patients experienced significant complications, these early conversations provided important guidance to families and physicians, helping to ease the difficult decisions.

It may be noted in passing that such conversations are probably not as common as they should be. As observed in a study by Goldstein and coworkers [30], implantable cardioverter defibrillators can prolong a death process uncomfortably and sometimes needlessly, yet physicians discussed the possibility of deactivating the implantable cardioverter defibrillators in only 27 of 100 cases.

Reflections

Early trials of surgically implanted devices pose a variety of distinctive issues. Often these trials are not technically "research," yet they involve substantial levels of innovation, experimentation, and iterative change. Probably the most important single response must be enhanced communication. Investigators need to share questions, problems, and information with each other; with the corporation that developed and may modify the device; and, above all, with patients and families who need to understand the uncertainties and hazards, not just the excitement, of the adventure on which they are to embark. With proactive thought and care, those issues can be managed in ethically sound ways.

Acknowledgments

The author acknowledges with gratitude the very helpful comments provided on earlier drafts by Robert Sade, MD, Edward Berger, PhD, Dorothy Vawter, PhD, and Martin McKneally, MD.

References

[1] ABIOMED. http://www.abiomed.com/products/heart_replacement/product_details.cfm. Accessed July 24, 2005.
[2] Frazier OH, Dowling RD, Gray LA, et al. The total artificial heart: where we stand. Cardiology 2004;101:117–21.
[3] Dowling RD, Gray Jr LA, Etoch SW, et al. Initial experience with the AbioCor implantable replacement heart system. J Thorac Cardiovasc Surg 2004;127:131–41.
[4] Dowling RD, Gray Jr LA, Etoch SW, et al. The AbioCor implantable replacement heart. Ann Thorac Surg 2003;75(6 Suppl):S93–9.
[5] ABIOMED. www.abiomed.com. Accessed July 24, 2005.
[6] ABIOMED. http://www.abiomed.com/products/heart_replacement/indications.cfm. Accessed July 24, 2005.
[7] Gil G. Abiomed knew of membrane problem: Christerson, others decided against new heart. Louisville Courier-Journal February 11, 2003. http://www.courier-journal.com/localnews/2003/02/11/ke021103s364449.htm. Accessed February 11, 2003.
[8] Dow Jones Newswires. ABIOMED completes clinical, engineering, mfg analyses after death of AbioCor patient. October 21, 2004. http://online.wsj.com/article/0,BT_CO_20041021_009075,00.html. Accessed October 21, 2004.
[9] Macklin R. Ethical implications of surgical experiments. Am Coll Surg Bull 1985;70:2–5.
[10] Miller FG. Sham surgery: an ethical analysis. Am J Bioethics 2003;3:41–8.
[11] Macklin R. The ethical problems with sham surgery in clinical research. N Engl J Med 1999;341:992–6.
[12] Freeman TB, Vawter DE, Leaverton PE, et al. Use of placebo surgery in controlled trials of a cellular-based therapy for Parkinson's disease. N Engl J Med 1999;341:988–91.
[13] London AJ, Kadane JB. Placebos that harm: sham surgery controls in clinical trials. Statistical Methods in Medical Research 2002;11:413–27.
[14] Black N. Evidence-based surgery: a passing fad? World J Surg 1999;23:789–93.
[15] Witkin KB. Clinical trials in development and marketing of medical devices. In: Witkin KB, editor. Clinical evaluation of medical devices: principles and case studies. Totowa (NJ): Humana Press; 1998. p. 3–21.
[16] Ramsey SD, Luce BR, Deyo R, et al. The limited state of technology assessment for medical devices: facing the issues. Am J Managed Care 1998;4:SP188–99.
[17] McKneally MF. Ethical problems in surgery: innovation leading to unforeseen complications. World J Surg 1999;23:786–8.
[18] McKneally MF. A bypass for the institutional review board: reflections on the Cleveland Clinic study of the Batista operation. J Thorac Cardiovasc Surg 2001;121:837–9.
[19] Grunkemeier GL. Clinical studies of prosthetic heart valves using historical controls. In: Witkin KB, editor. Clinical evaluation of medical devices: principles and case studies. Totowa (NJ): Humana Press; 1998. p. 83–102.
[20] Neugebauer E, Troidl H, Spangenberger W, et al. Conventional versus laparoscopic cholecystectomy and the randomized controlled trial. Br J Surg 1991;78:150–4.
[21] 45 CFR §46.102(d).
[22] Morreim EH. Litigation in clinical research: malpractice doctrines versus research realities. J Law Med Ethics 2004;32:474–84.
[23] Morreim EH. End-stage heart disease, high-risk research, and competence to consent: the case of the AbioCor artificial heart. Perspect Biol Med, in press.
[24] Altman LA. How to assist failing hearts? New questions emerge. New York Times November 20, 2001.
[25] Appelbaum PS, Roth LH, Lidz C. The therapeutic misconception: informed consent in psychiatric research. Int J Law Psychiatry 1982;5:319–29.

[26] Appelbaum PS, Roth LH, Lidz CW, et al. False hopes and best data: consent to research and the therapeutic misconception. Hastings Cent Rep 1987;17:20–4.

[27] DeVries WC. The physician, the media, and the 'spectacular' case. JAMA 1988;259:886–90.

[28] Kaptchuk TJ, Goldman P, Stone DA, et al. Do medical devices have enhanced placebo effects? J Clin Epidemiol 2000;53:786–92.

[29] *Goodman v United States*, 298 F3d 1048 (9th Cir 2002).

[30] Goldstein NE, Lampert R, Bradley E, et al. Management of implantable cardioverter defibrillators in end-of-life care. Ann Intern Med 2004;141:835–8.

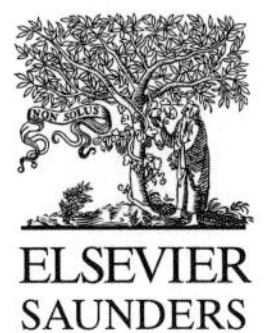

ELSEVIER
SAUNDERS

Thorac Surg Clin 15 (2005) 565–583

THORACIC
SURGERY
CLINICS

Cumulative Index 2005

Note: Page numbers of article titles are in **boldface** type.

A

1547-4127/05/$ – see front matter
doi:10.1016/S1547-4127(05)00099-X

B

C

D

E

F

G

J

K

L

P

R

U

V

W

X

Changing Your Address?

Make sure your subscription changes too! When you notify us of your new address, you can help make our job easier by including an exact copy of your Clinics label number with your old address (see illustration below.) This number identifies you to our computer system and will speed the processing of your address change. Please be sure this label number accompanies your old address and your corrected address—you can send an old Clinics label with your number on it or just copy it exactly and send it to the address listed below.

We appreciate your help in our attempt to give you continuous coverage. Thank you.

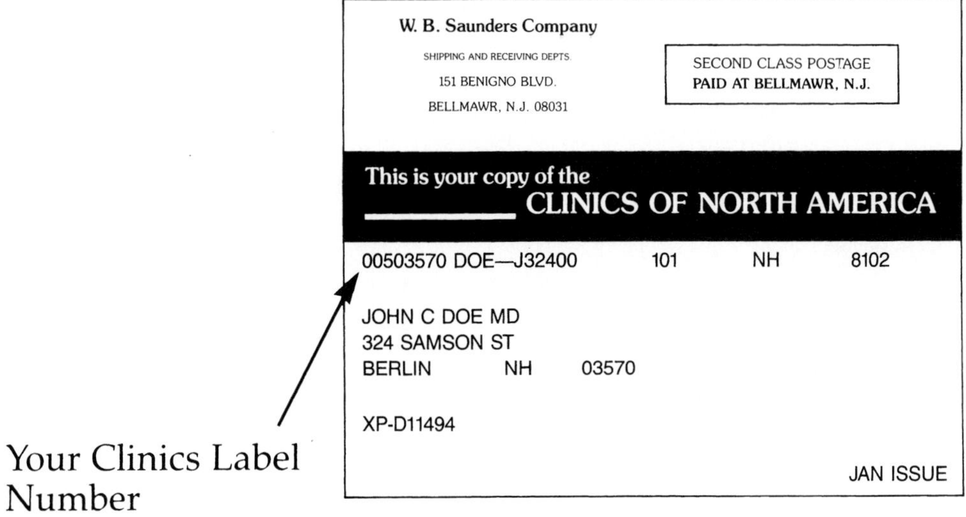

Your Clinics Label Number

Copy it exactly or send your label along with your address to:
W.B. Saunders Company, Customer Service
Orlando, FL 32887-4800
Call Toll Free 1-800-654-2452

Please allow four to six weeks for delivery of new subscriptions and for processing address changes.

United States Postal Service

Statement of Ownership, Management, and Circulation

1. Publication Title	2. Publication Number	3. Filing Date
Thoracic Surgery Clinics	1 5 4 7 - 4 1 2 7	9/15/05
4. Issue Frequency	5. Number of Issues Published Annually	6. Annual Subscription Price
Feb, May, Aug, Nov	4	$175.00

7. Complete Mailing Address of Known Office of Publication (*Not printer*) (*Street, city, county, state, and ZIP+4*)

Elsevier, Inc.
6277 Sea Harbor Drive
Orlando, FL 32887-4800

Contact Person: Gwen C. Campbell
Telephone: 215-239-3685

8. Complete Mailing Address of Headquarters or General Business Office of Publisher (*Not printer*)

Elsevier, Inc., 360 Park Avenue South, New York, NY 10010-1710

9. Full Names and Complete Mailing Addresses of Publisher, Editor, and Managing Editor (*Do not leave blank*)

Publisher (*Name and complete mailing address*)

Tim Griswold, Elsevier, Inc., 1600 John F. Kennedy Blvd. Suite 1800, Philadelphia, PA 19103-2899

Editor (*Name and complete mailing address*)

Catherine Bewick, Elsevier, Inc., 1600 John F. Kennedy Blvd. Suite 1800, Philadelphia, PA 19103-2899

Managing Editor (*Name and complete mailing address*)

Heather Cullen, Elsevier, Inc., 1600 John F. Kennedy Blvd. Suite 1800, Philadelphia, PA 19103-2899

10. Owner (*Do not leave blank. If the publication is owned by a corporation, give the name and address of the corporation immediately followed by the names and addresses of all stockholders owning or holding 1 percent or more of the total amount of stock. If not owned by a corporation, give the names and addresses of the individual owners. If owned by a partnership or other unincorporated firm, give its name and address as well as those of each individual owner. If the publication is published by a nonprofit organization, give its name and address.*)

Full Name	Complete Mailing Address
Wholly owned subsidiary of	4520 East-West Highway
Reed/Elsevier, US holdings	Bethesda, MD 20814

11. Known Bondholders, Mortgagees, and Other Security Holders Owning or Holding 1 Percent or More of Total Amount of Bonds, Mortgages, or Other Securities. If none, check box → ☐ None

Full Name	Complete Mailing Address
N/A	

12. Tax Status (*For completion by nonprofit organizations authorized to mail at nonprofit rates*) (*Check one*)
The purpose, function, and nonprofit status of this organization and the exempt status for federal income tax purposes:
☐ Has Not Changed During Preceding 12 Months
☐ Has Changed During Preceding 12 Months (*Publisher must submit explanation of change with this statement*)

(*See Instructions on Reverse*)

PS Form **3526**, October 1999

13. Publication Title: Thoracic Surgery Clinics

14. Issue Date for Circulation Data Below: August 2005

15. Extent and Nature of Circulation		Average No. Copies Each Issue During Preceding 12 Months	No. Copies of Single Issue Published Nearest to Filing Date
a. Total Number of Copies (*Net press run*)		2083	1800
b. Paid and/or Requested Circulation	(1) Paid/Requested Outside-County Mail Subscriptions Stated on Form 3541. (*Include advertiser's proof and exchange copies*)	851	823
	(2) Paid In-County Subscriptions Stated on Form 3541 (*Include advertiser's proof and exchange copies*)		
	(3) Sales Through Dealers and Carriers, Street Vendors, Counter Sales, and Other Non-USPS Paid Distribution	300	357
	(4) Other Classes Mailed Through the USPS		
c. Total Paid and/or Requested Circulation [*Sum of 15b. (1), (2), (3), and (4)*] →		1151	1180
d. Free Distribution by Mail (*Samples, compliment-ary, and other free*)	(1) Outside-County as Stated on Form 3541	74	89
	(2) In-County as Stated on Form 3541		
	(3) Other Classes Mailed Through the USPS		
e. Free Distribution Outside the Mail (*Carriers or other means*)			
f. Total Free Distribution (*Sum of 15d. and 15e.*) →		74	89
g. Total Distribution (*Sum of 15c. and 15f.*) →		1225	1269
h. Copies not Distributed		858	531
i. Total (*Sum of 15g. and h.*) →		2083	1800
j. Percent Paid and/or Requested Circulation (*15c. divided by 15g. times 100*)		94%	93%

16. Publication of Statement of Ownership
☐ Publication required. Will be printed in the **November 2005** issue of this publication. ☐ Publication not required

17. Signature and Title of Editor, Publisher, Business Manager, or Owner

Jean M. Fanucci - Executive Director of Subscription Services — Date: 9/15/05

I certify that all information furnished on this form is true and complete. I understand that anyone who furnishes false or misleading information on this form or who omits material or information requested on the form may be subject to criminal sanctions (including fines and imprisonment) and/or civil sanctions (including civil penalties).

Instructions to Publishers

1. Complete and file one copy of this form with your postmaster annually on or before October 1. Keep a copy of the completed form for your records.
2. In cases where the stockholder or security holder is a trustee, include in items 10 and 11 the name of the person or corporation for whom the trustee is acting. Also include the names and addresses of individuals who are stockholders who own or hold 1 percent or more of the total amount of bonds, mortgages, or other securities of the publishing corporation. In item 11, if none, check the box. Use blank sheets if more space is required.
3. Be sure to furnish all circulation information called for in item 15. Free circulation must be shown in items 15d, e, and f.
4. Item 15h., Copies not Distributed, must include (1) newsstand copies originally stated on Form 3541, and returned to the publisher, (2) estimated returns from news agents, and (3), copies for office use, leftovers, spoiled, and all other copies not distributed.
5. If the publication had Periodicals authorization as a general or requester publication, this Statement of Ownership , Management, and Circulation must be published; it must be printed in any issue in October or, if the publication is not published during October, the first issue printed after October.
6. In item 16, indicate the date of the issue in which this Statement of Ownership will be published.
7. Item 17 must be signed.

Failure to file or publish a statement of ownership may lead to suspension of Periodicals authorization.

PS Form **3526**, October 1999 (*Reverse*)